Measured Meals

Measured Meals

Nutrition in America

Jessica J. Mudry

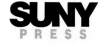

SUNY
PRESS

Published by
State University of New York Press, Albany

Printed in the United States of America

For information, contact State University of New York Press, Albany, NY
www.sunypress.edu

Production by Cathleen Collins
Marketing by Fran Keneston

Library of Congress Cataloging-in-Publication Data

Mudry, Jessica J., 1974–
  Measured meals : nutrition in America / Jessica J. Mudry.
    p. cm.
  Includes bibliographical references and index.
  ISBN 978-0-7914-9381-6 (hardcover : alk. paper)
    1. Nutrition—United States.   2. Nutrition policy—United States.   3. Diet—
United States.   4. Rhetoric.   I. Title.

  TX360.U6M83 2009
  613.20973—dc22   2008033400

                    10 9 8 7 6 5 4 3 2 1

For Eliot and Julien

Contents

Illustrations

Acknowledgments

Many people supported me through the process of crafting this book and I am indebted to their kindness. I feel forever owing to Joan Leach, a model scholar who asks important questions, and, in this case, made me ask important questions to get to the heart of this book. I owe an enormous amount to Jonathan Sterne. Jon is a brilliant man who made this project more insightful and well rounded by making me think about old things in new ways. I would like to thank Carrie Rentschler for being a spirited confidante who instilled confidence in my work, by instilling confidence in me. Jonathan Erlen, History of Medicine librarian at the University of Pittsburgh, was always a great resource, and someone who was always supportive of my work. Also, I would like to thank the University of Pittsburgh Mellon Fellowship program that supported me through much of the early research and writing of this book. I owe much to Larin McLaughlin at State University of New York Press for working so hard on behalf of this book. I would also like to thank the reviewers, in particular Katie LeBesco, who made excellent suggestions for improvements to the manuscript. Parts of chapter 2 have been published previously in *Food, Culture and Society*, 9, 1 (2006): 49–67, and are reprinted here by permission of Berg Publishers.

It is important to me to recognize here the support of my friends: Sarah Graham, Jillian Moncarz, and Kay Osmak. Our camaraderie carried me through much of the writing of this book. You are among the most patient, successful, and wonderful people I know. I owe special thanks to my Baba Sophie Vasileff, my maternal grandmother, whose life inspired this book, and who continues to cook without the aid of measuring cups, eat without counting calories, and love without condition. To my parents, Ben and Fran Mudry, I am forever indebted to your graciousness, your generosity, your support, and your love. It is from you that I learned the value of hard work, a value that underpins this entire project, and a value that I hope to be able to pass on to my own children. You are exceptional parents, outstanding grandparents, and I love you very much.

Finally, to my partner Robert Danisch, I owe you more than I could possibly articulate. I treasure your unfailing love, your boundless energy and optimism, your intelligence and wit, and your friendship. Without you, this book would be a muddled idea; indeed, so might I. Thank you for the clarity you provide to me, to us, and to our family, without fail, every day.

Introduction

Eating by Numbers

How Language Shapes Food and Eating

This book is about how language affects what we eat and how we eat. Over the past century, talking about food in terms of calories, vitamins, and serving sizes has become commonplace. These commonplaces have a history, and their history reveals their influence on America's relationship to food. As the science of nutrition marches on, producing more and more knowledge regarding the connection between diet and health, Americans seem increasingly confused about what to eat to stay healthy. How can we account for the increase in sound, scientific advice about the health benefits of diet and the concomitant increase in diseases related to diet? One way to answer this question is to consider how language figures food, eating, diet, and health. This is another way of saying that analyzing communicative practices can help better explain America's strained relationship to food.

On April 19, 2005, the Secretary of the United States Department of Agriculture (USDA) released MyPyramid, a new federal food guide designed to present "Steps to a Healthier You." MyPyramid aims to provide the "best" daily food choices for Americans, and represents the USDA's latest attempt to get Americans to listen to sound, scientific dietary advice. MyPyramid can be customized. When visiting the USDA website, a person can enter their age, gender, and activity level, and the pyramid will present the number of calories per day that person needs along with the number of ounces a day of each food group that would supply those calories.

MyPyramid follows a discursive framework of food guidance that has been around since the USDA's inception. In figuring the ideal national diet using calories, proportions, minutes, servings, and groups, the USDA deploys a language of quantification to describe food. This book recounts the development and effects of that language. Since its inception in 1862, the USDA's methods of research, documentation, and reporting have been guided by science. As a result, the way the USDA communicates ideas about "soils, grains, fruits, vegetables, and manures" (USDA, Congress Bill 249) has been in and through statistics and quantities. The first USDA food guide, published in 1917, initiates the use of a scientific and enumerated framework for understanding food. Almost one hundred years later, MyPyramid does not stray from the discursive course. In telling the history of this discursive course, I hope to show how and why a quantitative language of food and nutrition developed and the effects that it has had.

Discourses of science in general, and quantification in particular, have been around in a variety of forms for centuries. Quantification is one method for understanding, explaining, and analyzing. To impose order, coerce or control a complex world, quantification provides surety, distinction, and ease of manipulation of people, places, and things. In the past this order was established by systems of measurement for everything from grain to wool to arable land. Many goods that we measure according to the universal system of weights were first measured using arbitrary and often anthropomorphic systems of quantification. A "finger" of powder or a "hand" of honey scarcely resembles our abstract systems of metric or imperial measures of today. These systems, however, demonstrated the capacity for abstract quantitative thinking, in which the amount of an object became part of its qualitative property. This thinking also allowed for comparison between disparate objects. A journey, a noodle, and a bug could all be measured and compared by their length; an elephant, a bunch of bananas, and an atom could all be discussed and compared in terms of their weight. As federal nutrition guidance evolved with technologies like proximate analysis, the calorimeter, and X-ray crystallography a diet could be ordered, controlled, and understood through measurable factors: calories, fat grams, protein, and eventually vitamins, minerals, and amino acids. Organizations like the USDA now attempt to legislate a healthy diet by mandating quantities of foods based on measurable nutrients.

In order to trace the development and effects of this discourse of quantification, I analyze American federal food guides produced by the USDA over the last 100 years. Examining and interpreting American federal nutrition documentation reveals three important things. First, such an examination reveals how the science of nutrition developed in America:

what technologies researchers used, how they used them, and to what ends. Second, such an examination reveals how the *language* of nutrition evolved over time. And third, such an examination can demonstrate how language reframed, reshaped, and attempted to control what Americans were eating. In analyzing these documents, I am relying on concepts from contemporary rhetorical theory and the rhetoric of science. Such a framework can show how language works within discursive communities to make meaning and can elucidate how language coordinates social action.

In the light of my analysis of federal nutrition guidance, I argue that the use of a quantitative language to prescribe a "healthy" national diet is a failure. Understanding food through quantities and talking about food using a discourse of quantification undermines the sense of taste that is employed when we eat. This discourse is impoverished because it feeds certain human sensibilities only: rationality, reduction, and objectivity. The USDA encourages the "healthy" eater to categorize herself based on the number of calories per day her body requires and to eat particular quantities of food to fill that caloric need. Policy that employs this kind of language in attempts to rationalize the sensibilities of the human body is doomed to fail until it can supplement a discourse of quantification with alternative languages that speak to the subject of the body not the object of the body. Understanding food through discourses of tradition, culture, geography, history, and taste are some of the qualitative manners of communicating health and well-being that can supplement and complement a quantitative discourse. As it stands, the paradox of more sound, scientific advice regarding health and nutrition along with the simultaneous increases in diet-related diseases is best described as a problem of communication. Moreover, this is a problem grounded in the use of a particular language.

The purpose of this book is, first, to recount the development of a scientific and quantitative discourse regarding food, nutrition, and health over the last hundred years. Second, my goal in recounting such a history is to explain why that discourse emerged in the way that it did and what effect it has had. This kind of rhetorical history grounds the larger argument that American nutrition policy is incomplete or inadequate because it distorts judgments about eating, discounts other knowledge claims regarding health, and unfairly reimagines the nature of food. Such an argument is part of a larger conversation regarding the history of science, broadly, and the history of nutrition, narrowly. Historians of science are at their best when they attend to the function of language in generating knowledge claims, but historians of food and nutrition have often overlooked this very feature of scientific work. It is my hope that a rhetorical perspective on food and nutrition will accommodate for this oversight. In the rest of this introduction, I will tell the broader story of the role of science and quantification in American public life and show how this book adds to that story. I will also show how histories of nutrition overlook the importance of quantitative language in framing health issues and attempt to redress that oversight by positioning my argument within other work on the rhetoric of science. And finally, I will outline the significance of my argument for America's relationship with food and point to the general effects the use of quantitative language has had.

Science and Quantification in American Public Life

For over 2000 years, numbers, measurements, and quantities have been the defining characteristics of things civilized, refined, and enlightened. All three monotheistic religions, Islam, Christianity, and Judaism, make reference to codes of conduct bound up in measuring actions, weighing consequences, and exacting and meting equally with others. Deuteronomy 25:13–15 (revised standard version) proclaims:

> You shall not have in your bag two kinds of weights, a large and a small. You shall not have in your house two kinds of measures, a large and a small. A full and just weight you shall have, a full and just measure you shall have; that your days may be prolonged in the land which the Lord your God gives you.

The "perfect and just measure," an exact standard, was the means to longevity, and perfection and justice were bound up in measure. Measurement gave a means for comparison, a resolution to argument, and a system of living. Counting, comparing, and measuring are components of the human practice of quantifying.

It was often the case that measured quantities were on display in public places like the market or the town hall. To ensure their longevity and incontrovertibility, quantities of weight and length were cast in metal or stone. Often, these measures carried the mark or seal of a government or religious official to prevent public debate over their accuracy. Exact measurements, represented by numbers and established by the government, relieved the public of having to rely on personal judgment for determining quantities. Quantities ended conversation, resolved disputes, and silenced public dissent. The guarantee of the immutability of measures, quantities, and standards provided a modicum of social order and control (Kula, 1986; Crosby, 1997; Menninger, 1969; Frängsmyr, 1990). Exactitude replaced personal opinion and helped to craft a particular quantitative discourse that acted to control and organize human relationships to objects of use. Bound up in the knowledge of quantification and measures, and their standardization, is an understanding of, and respect for, civilization, social stability, and social control (Porter, 1986).

Stated measures and quantities allowed people to discuss and trade amounts of incongruent entities without the shadiness of opinions. Such measures, therefore, abated private disputes by deferring to public and impartial standards. In addition, quantification provided a strategy for extending the burgeoning rationalistic and objective character of modern society. The use of quantities and measurements in society aided the assumption that numbers could "remove values from anything," and by removing values, numbers could serve as the grammar for a new language for thinking about the world absent adjectives, adverbs, and other descriptive qualifiers (Cohen, 1999, p. 46).

John Ziman (1978) calls the language of numbers "unambiguous communication," and it was the unambiguous nature of this language that made it the choice for the communication of science (p. 11). Scientists sought a formalized language, one that could transmit knowledge with "perfect precision and overwhelming certitude." Thus, the ultimate step, claims Ziman, is to "transform it [science] into *mathematics* . . . the urge to express all scientific knowledge in mathematical terms is an elementary consequence of our model of science" (p. 12). Given this kind of communication, "scientists who are familiar with such a system of definitions and axioms can send each other unambiguous messages" (p. 13). Science relies on quantification to encourage and acknowledge certain sureties. A calorie is universally recognized by the scientific community as the amount of heat needed to raise the temperature of one gram of water from 14.5 °C to 15.5 °C. Fixing this value allows scientists to talk in terms of calories and to compare and contrast amounts of heat given off by engines, supernovas, and people. This language of numbers is the bedrock upon which much scientific communication happens and even acts to define a discipline as science. The keynote speaker at a conference on the history of quantification in the sciences proclaimed: "once a new discipline has developed a mathematical discourse, it has almost immediately laid claim, at least in the language of its most enthusiastic disciples, to the significant status—science" (Woolf, 1961, p. 3).

The understanding of food encouraged by the U.S. government is part of the broader American fascination with science, standards, and quantification. In *No Other Gods: On Science and American Social Life*, historian Charles Rosenberg (1976) shows that during the 17th and 18th centuries science played a prominent role in the discourses of the American colonial elite. Among the early American elite, an understanding of science and medicine was as fundamental to a well-rounded curriculum as Latin and theology. Rosenberg argues that, for the most part, science worked itself seamlessly into the fabric of American social discourse. Social order and American social structure depended greatly on the acceptance of knowledge produced by "men of learning" (p. 3). An efficient democratic government required methods of quantification, order, and standards. To reject this scientific knowledge was to reject order and stability in society.

Science completed its rise in the hierarchy of American values around the turn of the 20th century, and as it assumed a more significant place in American life, it shaped and influenced the communication of social norms. Many historians of science point to the period of urbanization and industrialization in the late 1800s to 1920s as the era facilitating America's political and cultural acceptance of science, order, and social standards. The idea that it was always better, in cases of difficulty, to have clear standards than to depend on personal judgment became important in developing a public trust in numbers (Porter, 1995). This American respect for, and trust in, numbers is central to understanding a language of quantification, how it works in American public discourse, and why it became a default mode of communication about food. In any case, it is clear that science played an increasingly important role in American public policy in the 20th century. Therefore, it should be no surprise that the USDA relied on scientific knowledge to craft policies regarding health, diet, and nutrition.

Over the course of the 20th century the alignment between science and government became ever more complex and intricate, and it continued to rely on an expanding discourse of quantification. This alignment was facilitated by the professionalization of science and the relationship between research universities and government. Many historians have told the story of professionalization in an effort to track the effects of science on American public life (Balogh, 1991; Wiebe, 1967; Oleson and Voss, 1979). Most notably, Thomas Haskell (2000) shows how specialization generated authority for a class of professionals, and Roger Geiger (2004) tells part of the latter story of how the relationship between government and science was fostered by research universities. In what follows, I will show how the USDA's use of a discourse of quantification relied explicitly on the evidence generated by experiment stations at American universities. This evidence was a product of professionals and specialists making claims to authority by virtue of a scientific ethos. As such, this story fits into broader trends identified by Haskell, Geiger, and others. In *The Social Transformation of American Medicine*, Paul Starr (1982) tells a more specific story about the history of health and medicine in the United

States. This is also a story of professionalization, specialization, and the consolidation of authority in the light of expertise and bureaucracy. Starr goes further to show how economics had a hand in the transformation of medicine. All of these histories have made tremendous advances in our understanding of the social constitution of scientific practices and in tracking the implications of those practices for American public life.

But when historians point to the relationship between science and a discourse of quantification, between professionalization and science, or between government and science, the implied assumption, that scientific language does not distort and cannot be misinterpreted, is almost never critically tested. This assumption relies on a broader misunderstanding of communication as "conduit," an assumption employed in many places and toward many different ends (Ortony, 1993, pp. 284–324). Language is almost never thought of as constitutive of scientific practice or integral to the development of scientific knowledge. In the light of Thomas Kuhn's (1970/1996) *Structure of Scientific Revolutions*, recent debates in the philosophy of science, social epistemology, and the rhetoric of science have opened several critical questions regarding the relationship between language and ontology, epistemology, and ethics (Fuller, 1988; Gross, 1996; Gross and Keith, 1997; Bazerman, 1988; Latour and Woolgar, 1986). Often work in these fields relies on examples from the history of science to track the role of language in the discovery and dissemination of new knowledge. Such work will, for example, point out specific metaphors, analogies, and metonymies that operate alongside a quantitative discourse to suggest that language can never be reduced to numbers and that science consistently engages in acts of persuasion. Rarely is a discourse of quantification itself understood as metaphoric or metonymic, but, as I will show later, quantification tropes the objects being described. It is my intention to bring some of the insights from the rhetoric of science to bear on a particular example of the history of science in American public policy. Such a move, I argue, is necessary if we are to understand the full effects of science on American public life. I hope that this more critical history will further develop the implications of the work of Ziman, Rosenberg, Haskell, Geiger, Starr, and others by illuminating the way that linguistic choices can constrain, limit, refigure, reimagine, reshape, or redefine our relationship to food.

Food, Nutrition, and Health as Rhetorics of Science

To call this kind of history a rhetorical history requires that I explain what I mean by *rhetoric*, broadly, and the *rhetoric of science*, specifically. The word "rhetoric" has well-known negative connotations. But recent years have seen a resurgence in the study of rhetoric throughout the humanities (Nelson, Megill, and McCloskey, 1987). This resurgence is guided by a view of rhetoric as a kind of communicative practice. More specifically, it is a communicative practice that seeks persuasion, is planned, considers audiences, shapes knowledge, and coordinates social action (Hauser, 2002; Herrick, 1997). The purpose of rhetoric is to "influence human choices" through the management of symbols (Hauser, 2002, p. 3). The study of rhetoric, therefore, includes a concern with the methods used in constructing persuasive discourse and a concern with the manner in which "symbolic performances influence practical choices" (p. 12). A rhetorical history considers the ways in which persuasive discourse has been shaped over a long period of time, and how, in the past, symbolic performances have influenced, or attempted to influence, practical choices. This is what I mean when I call this history of food and nutrition a rhetorical history.

In the light of work by Alan Gross (1996, 2006), Marcello Pera (1994), and others (McCloskey, 1998; Halliday and Martin, 1993), scientific discourse has been analyzed as a set of symbolic practices that seek persuasion, consider audiences, shape knowledge, and coordinate social action, and thus is a form of rhetoric in action. From this perspective one of the most intractable questions has concerned whether, or to what extent, rhetoric is constitutive of knowledge. In what follows, I argue that it is and show why and how it is. Other rhetoricians of science make a similar argument by pointing to the way that analogy, metaphor, metonymy, and other stylistic devices are integral to the invention of scientific knowledge (Fahnestock, 1999; Graves, 2005). My focus, however, is on a discourse of quantification, itself, as a stylistic device that tropes and refigures the objects it describes. As such, I use some of the techniques provided by the rhetoric of science, but I try to extend that work by accounting for the rhetoricity of quantification.

Because pure objectivity lies at the heart of quantification, it claims to defy social and cultural constraints and immunity from sociological analysis or criticism (Bloor, 1991). One can measure out two pints of milk, and see that this volume is more than one pint and less than three. This measurement is immune from emotional or subjective arguments. Once these measurements are used to create relationships in the marketplace, selling milk, for example, becomes an exercise in calculation. How much milk I can purchase for one dollar becomes a comparative activity: where can I buy more and spend the least? Moreover, numbers abet the quantification of the personal value of quality. One milk may be better than another because it costs less or because it is fortified with extra vitamin D, thus forcing questions such as: How much am I willing to spend on a quality product? Is a small quantity worth more, if the quality is better? One particular result of numeration is its exploitation of numbers, statistics, and measurements to valorize and legitimate inferential and qualitative experiences. The use of this numerated and measured discourse conflates and confuses qualities and quantities—this is one of the most important consequences of the use of a discourse of quantification.

To define a *discourse of quantification*, then, is to amalgamate the notions of discourse, quantity, and the social resonance of science, measurements, numbers, and amounts. I use the word "discourse" to highlight the organized and structured nature of scientific language, and to point to the importance of viewing language as a form of social practice. Most importantly, contemporary scholars have shown that discourse produces multiple effects, not all of which are intended. The basis of the persuasiveness and power of numbers, quantities, and measures lies with the notion of objectivity, truth, and freedom from personal opinion and error. For example, John Ziman argues: "The primary foundation for belief in science is the widespread impression that it is *objective*. The objectivity of scientific knowledge resides in its being a social construct, not owing its origin to any particular individual but created cooperatively and communally" (p. 107). Historically, objectivity has meant the rule of the law, and the subordination of personal interests and prejudices to public standards. Understanding a discourse within which objectivity begins to take on these meanings points to the unintended consequences of social practices that employ such a discourse.

From my perspective, a discourse of quantification, as a social practice, is a form of persuasive communication. It exhorts certain actions and thoughts (intentionally or not), and forms the basis for particular epistemologies. It is a discourse that employs numbers, amounts, degrees, or standards to create knowledge. These numbers outline a kind of vocabulary that dictates how this discourse operates and upon whom. When we communicate with quantities, there is a direction to our discourse and this direction limits the choices available to us. A discourse of quantification is a selectively silencing discourse. It encourages certain interactions and eliminates others because only certain ideas, arguments, and topoi can operate within it.

The concept of quantity has no content of its own. It relies on material things to bring it into existence. Accordingly, quantity works as a commonplace, or topic, by suggesting lines of argument that rely on objectivity and materiality. It is within this framework that the USDA constructed arguments about what to eat. The project of inventing things to say about food was guided by the topic of quantification. To extend this line of thinking, Gerard Hauser (2002) claims that "rhetorical invention consists in the act of finding suasive sayables by thinking of a subject in terms of *topoi*" (p. 112). Reading USDA food guides illustrates rhetorical invention in these terms because food is articulated using quantities, and attempts to establish discursive control of human interaction with food are quantitative. This is not unusual; quantification and science were fundamental and frequently used persuasive topoi throughout the 20th century. Richard Weaver (1995) attests to this. He claims that the word "science" obtains its "rhetorical character" from its association with "the undiluted essence of knowledge" and the "facts" that science purports to generate through its "method" (pp. 215–216).

Historically, quantification and the objectivity it confers, provided a cornerstone for a political philosophy that connoted a dispassionate means for generating a set of public rules. Ted Porter (1995) outlines the history of this political philosophy:

> Strict quantification, through measurement, counting, and calculation, is among the most credible strategies for rendering nature or society objective. . . . The ideal of objectivity is a political as well as a scientific one. Objectivity means the rule of law, not of men. It implies the subordination of personal interests and prejudices to public standards . . . quantification for public as well as scientific purposes has generally been allied to a spirit of rigor. (p. 74)

The USDA relied on this "spirit of rigor" and the "rule of law" to create trust in their authority and to help cast the notion of quality food into quantitative terms. Because quantification negated the subjective voice, it seemed a natural conduit for a government body to deliver information and create knowledge.

The USDA also used a discourse of quantification as an apparatus of epistemology. As Scott Montgomery (1996) writes, "What sort of faith, then, might we say seems to beat at the heart of this discourse? Simply this: that language can be made a form of technology, a device able to contain and transfer knowledge *without touching it*" (p. 2). A discourse of quantification is a generative mechanism. It gives rise to arguments, agendas, lines of thought, and bases for knowledge production within its own discursive bounds. Its objectivity bolsters its authority and is privileged by the USDA as the only discourse useful in crafting new knowledge of quality food. As Alan Gross (1996) puts it in *The Rhetoric of Science*: "[S]cientific prose generally excepts any device that shifts the reader's attention from the world that language creates to language itself as a resource for creating worlds" (p. 43).

What does it mean, then, to understand food, nutrition, and health as rhetorics of science? First, and perhaps most importantly, such a perspective implies that we see these concepts not as stable, secure, and closed objects or bodies of knowledge but as dynamic, changing, historically and culturally constituted artifacts. The concepts of food, nutrition, and health are a product of social practices, and the use of language is one of the critical social practices that produce these concepts. In other words, food, nutrition, and health do not precede language but are conceptually constituted by linguistic choices. Second, science functions as a persuasive practice in the constitution of these concepts. It highlights, selects, and points to some features of each while neglecting, ignoring, and overlooking other features. Science, by producing a language game within which food, nutrition, and health are defined, controls, orders, and organizes what can and cannot be said about those concepts and regulates the relationships people can have with those concepts. Third, the knowledge that we have about food, nutrition, and health are products of how those concepts are figured by a discourse of science. Attending to the ways in which language figures and refigures these concepts allows one to track the effects of this language. By studying food, nutrition, and health as rhetorics of science I am most interested in recounting and explaining those effects.

Figuring Food and the American Eater

At the center of a rhetorical approach to the history of food and nutrition is an account of how language figures food and eating. This is just what is missing in histories of nutrition and other analyses of America's relationship to food. For example, Walter Gratzer's (2005) *Terrors of the Table* is full of interesting anecdotes from the history of nutrition, but, as a biophysicist, Gratzer never challenges the underlying assumption that science is a mirror of reality and scientific evidence is sound and inherently beneficial in countless ways. Nor does Gratzer even wonder about language or test the limits or effects of communication through quantities. Cultural criticisms of food do not make a move to analyze the language of nutrition either. Marion Nestle's (2002) excellent *Food Politics* delivers a thorough critique of the influence of politics and industry on dietary advice. But Nestle never critiques the language of nutrition itself, and instead assumes that nutritionists are just producing more sound research that the public never quite accepts or understands. I agree with Nestle that politics and economics are deeply influential factors in crafting dietary advice, but that advice is always couched in the terms of a particular discourse. To overlook the historical development of that discourse is to miss how language figures food and eating.

To claim that language is figurative is to suggest that the use of stylistic devices creates associations between otherwise disparate things. It is also to argue that the language we choose to describe, for example, food, eating, and eaters, is constitutive of the meaning of those concepts and what we might know about those concepts. I suggest throughout that quantification is a figurative device. This implies that using numbers to describe foods creates associations between foods and other concepts that are not immediately referred to in the name of a food. Furthermore, figures of speech (including quantitative figures) play an important role in the invention of knowledge. This is not necessarily a new argument (Graves, 2005), but the claim that numbers perform this function is a new twist on this argument. To say that language figures food, eating, and the eater is to suggest that a discourse of quantification does not mirror the world as it actually is but that it invents a world within which certain sentences are true or false, certain behaviors are beneficial and harmful, and certain courses of action are recommended.

Four critical arguments result from this perspective. First, in the process of figuring food a new reality is certified by a new language. This is an ontological argument. To claim that a glass of milk is 150 calories is to call a particular reality into existence; a reality that did not exist prior to the use of the calorimeter and the generation of numbers that could describe milk in such terms. In this case, milk's caloric content is more real than its color, flavor, or smell. Because calories are a scientifically tested standard, they are useful in certifying the superiority of one reality over others. No one can see, touch, taste, or smell a calorie, but we all know that calories are real and an inherent property of all foods. The invention and use of a discourse of quantification, therefore, refigures food by making real new qualities of foods and suggesting that those qualities are the most important. The first major effect of a discourse of quantification is the invention and certification of a new reality, and given this effect, food *is* no longer what it used to *be*.

Second, a new epistemology is generated on the basis of this new reality. This new epistemology is responsible for ordering, controlling, and organizing the relationship between food and the people who consume food and their health. The new reality certified by a discourse of quantification obviously lends itself to a quantitative epistemology. As more numbers are generated to describe food, those numbers are put into relationship with one another in order to develop a way of knowing what is best to eat and why. The explanations offered by this new epistemology also countermand other types of knowledge claims. For example, knowledge about calories and vitamins is far more important than knowledge about seasonality and taste. Knowing about this new reality becomes a method of dismissing other, less rational, less sophisticated, less esoteric, or less professional knowledge claims.

Third, within this new ontology and epistemology all qualities become quantities. Invariably, qualitative questions of "good" and "bad" become inextricably linked to the language of quantity. In other words, good and bad are now products of calculation, not social determination. Throughout the course of the 20th century, the invention of numeric markers sought to replace any other available markers for determining whether or not a food was good. This is another way in which taste, seasonality, and culture are removed from conversations about food. Such alternative discourses cannot produce sufficient, rational evidence as to why a food might be good or bad.

Fourth, the eater is refigured as ethically incomplete. Underpinning the USDA's food guides are imagined audiences, or groups of Americans, that become the foci of reception of the discourse. "America," "Americans," or "eaters," as I often refer to them, are not actual samples of the population or people, but rather signifiers that are invented by the USDA. The formation of these groups, and their numeric management by the USDA, represent a kind of "cultural subject," produced and organized by policy and discourse. Toby Miller (1993), in *The Well-Tempered Self*, explains that the "cultural subject" is a fictional entity that is "governed through institutions and discourses" (p. ix). "Cultural subjects" are products of policy, dreamed up to represent populations whose behavior can be managed, remedied, or trained by discourses. In this project, the American eater is a cultural subject that is fabricated by the USDA to represent the heterogeneous mass of the American population. The USDA food guides, and much of the early nutrition research performed in the USDA-sanctioned labs, parses out this eater by sex, age, race, caloric needs, geography, and occupation. Though eating, tastes, and pleasure derived from food are largely cultural, experiential, and geographical, the USDA manages this disparity using a discourse of quantification.

A discourse of quantification, because it can be used to manage, group, and control both information and individuals who are implicated by that information, acts as an ideal milieu for the production of cultural subjects. By inscribing what Miller calls "ethical incompleteness," or a qualitative judgment upon the character of the person based on their adherence to policy initiatives, the USDA makes Americans and eaters a collective available for manipulation. The argument is that this collective can see their incompleteness in federal policy and attempt to remedy it or complete themselves using the discourse of the policy. A discourse of quantification makes achieving this completion easy, because achievement is not contained in subjective, or hard-to-define, political ideals. Completion for the American eater comes from abiding by nutritional numbers, eating enough, in moderation, more, or less, and by measuring themselves against numeric standards, the creation of which defines various cultural subjects. The USDA, through its early experiments on food and human metabolism, its food guides and their messages, and through the creation of norms and standards, manages publics by having them compare themselves to these externally generated numbers. Miller calls these guiding messages "technologies of governance" (p. xiii). These technologies, which may include everything from a calorimeter to a food guide to a pictorial representation of a good meal, help imprint ethical incompleteness upon the eater. The USDA's ideal, complete, and normal eater is numerate and well versed in a discourse of quantification. The ideal (but fictional) eater heeds nutritional advice, reads food labels and food guides, and compares his or her own food intake with what is normal for his or her USDA-defined demographic. This eater does not say things like "Broccoli isn't good," because the USDA eaters' bases for judging broccoli are folic acid content, fiber, or vitamin C, not whether they like the taste of broccoli.

Just as Miller does not find or interrogate "real people" in his investigations of public policy and governmentality, I have neither sought nor analyzed the specific reception of USDA food guides by actual subjects. Instead, the purpose of this work is to point to the effects, limits, and inadequacies of a discourse of quantification—its inability to know, in all its fullness, the place of food in American culture. By inventing "a kind of well-tempered self" the USDA clearly illustrates its incapacity for addressing the human and subjective facets of food and eating. A cultural subject is the only kind of subject available to a discourse of quantification because it is the only subject that avails itself to easy control, manipulation, and normalization.

These four critical effects ground the broad claim that quantification attempts to control what can be communicated about food, what can be known about food, and what food can represent. In employing a discourse of quantification, the USDA groups and normalizes people, thus organizing and ordering people's relationship to food. We see this in early dietary experiments, in USDA food guides, and in critiques of those guides. This order and organization issues from a discourse's ability to control how and what people know. In addition, a discourse of quantification is taxonomic. Numbers classify and differentiate because they represent discrete values. Food guides, for example, use numbers of nutrients to create food groups, as well as to determine the goodness or badness of foods. In *Writing Science*, M. A. K. Halliday (1993) addresses the ability of scientific language to organize our epistemological relationships:

> The biggest single demand that was explicitly made on a language of science was that it should be effective in constructing technical taxonomies. . . . Unlike commonsense knowledge, which can tolerate—indeed, depends on—compromises, contradictions and indeterminacies of all kinds, scientific knowledge as it was then coming into being needed to be organized around systems of technical concepts arranged in strict hierarchies of kinds and parts. (p. 6)

Using a discourse of quantification to order our relationship to food makes the management of this relationship easier for the administrative body of the USDA (Wise, 1995, p. 5). Food guides focused on systems of technical concepts and encouraged eaters to be concerned with what they were eating, not how they were eating. But these guides were never able to make America healthier according to the standards of health implied within the guides. By many standards, Americans are healthier now than they were 100 years ago. But official dietary advice has consistently invoked the promise of a healthier America in the light of new evidence about diet-related disease (by which I mean a whole range of problems from heart disease to type-2 diabetes). Thus the ever-shifting conception of health implied in these documents seems to be, ironically, an unachievable reality and an unrecognizable goal. With an ever-expanding capacity for measuring aspects of health, it seems that these quantitative standards indicate how increasingly unhealthy we are. But this might not be the case at all. A discourse of quantification wants an American public that is quantifiably healthier, but never seems capable of producing such a public.

If a discourse of quantification could not make America healthier by its own terms, it did facilitate a specific form of judgment. By judgment I mean functional ways to define values of good, bad, or normal. Judging food is no longer a question of flavor, taste, region, sensation, or season, but instead it is now a function of comparisons, charts, counting, and analyzing. A good meal contains 5 grams of fiber, a bad snack has more than 10 grams of sugar, and a normal serving size is 5 ounces. A discourse of quantification gives the eater and the USDA a common language thereby giving policy-makers easy access to patterns of food consumption, and providing both the eater and the government with the means to judge food. Measurement is not "simply a link to theory, but a technology for managing events" (Porter, 1995, p. 72). And in managing events we judge ourselves, our food, and our eating patterns by the available numbers and nothing more. From this discourse, we get a normal eater who practices self-judgment.

I will expand on each of these implications in the following chapters. In chapter 1, I show how the USDA founded and sanctioned experiment stations to generate scientific knowledge regarding food and nutrition and how Wilbur Atwater was able to determine the caloric value of specific foods. In chapters 2 and 3 I read USDA food guides to show how a discourse of quantification was used to attempt to influence dietary choices. In chapter 4, I analyze critiques of the USDA advice and show how those critiques are also embedded within a discourse of quantification. And in chapter 5, I point to the authority of history, geography, and experience as grounds for a discourse of taste. Such a discourse of taste points to one way for remedying the failures of the USDA. America's relationship with food has been altered by the invention and use of a discourse of quantification. Thus, each of these chapters tells the story of how and why this relationship was constituted in the way that it was.

What Should We Eat?

Over the course of the 20th century this question has become enormously complex. Government-sanctioned dietary advice attempts to answer the "should question" by reducing a food to its nutritional portfolio and determining whether or not that nutritional portfolio is good for one's health. The identification and quantification of a food's nutritional portfolio has driven the invention of an American culinary tradition and helped remake the structure of the entire food economy (Pollan, 2006). In addition, it has contributed to the creation of what Michael Pollan (2008) and Gyorgy Scrinis (2008) have called "nutritionism." Nutritionism and nutrition are not the same. Adding the *ism* suggests an ideology and not a scientific subject. An ideology is a comprehensive vision of the world that organizes experiences into a kind of common sense. This form of common sense is supported by a set of unexamined assumptions that make an ideology's values hard to critique, or even identify. The major, common sense assumptions behind nutritionism are that the hidden chemical elements, and the quantities of those elements, of a food are its most important features and that understanding these hidden chemical constituents will inevitably improve our health. The deepest implication of this ideology and these common sense assumptions is that answering the "should question" by anything other than quantitative/scientific criteria is a mistake. In that case, all other claims to authority or knowledge, all other attempts to answer the "should question" in terms of geography, culture, tradition, taste, and so forth, are, at best, misleading and, at worst, dangerous.

The history of the emergence of this common sense view of food and eating is inextricably tied to the development of a discourse of quantification. Perhaps more importantly, however, the emergence of this common sense view coincides with the erosion of culture, tradition, and taste as arbiters of eating habits, along with the erosion of qualitative assessments of health. It also happens to coincide with the increasing incidence of diet-related disease. By its own standards, it seems that nutritionism has failed to promote public health, its single, most important goal. It has, however, succeeded in rewarding specific companies with enormous profits and remaking the food-supply chain and reimagining what's for sale at the grocery store. Some might contend that it has also succeeded in causing unparalleled environmental degradation and great ecological harm. The story of quantification is intimately bound to stories about the functionalization of food, the invention of processed foods, the use of chemistry and genetics for the alteration of food crops, new techniques of refining, preserving, and delivering nutrients to the body, and the massive success of the fast-food industry. But the hidden effect of the story of quantification, the hidden effect of nutritionism's reduction of food to its chemical components, is a loss of other forms of knowledge, other criteria for answering the "should question," or, in other words, the loss, or at least the erosion, of the richness and diversity of other reasons to eat and other kinds of assessments of health. According to Leslie Brenner (2000), America has lost, or perhaps never had, its gastronomy. The story of the role of quantification and nutrition science explains why and what the stakes are in that loss.

In *Meals to Come*, Warren Belasco (2006) recounts another, parallel aspect of this story. Although he does not relate his "history of the future of food" to the ideology of nutritionism, it is clear that the imaginings of the future of food that he recounts hinge on, and are committed to, the technological and scientific advancement of nutrition and agricultural science. The meal in a pill is perhaps the best illustration of the ideology of nutritionism from Belasco's history because it nicely demonstrates the reduction of food to its nutritional portfolio and the elimination of social eating practices (the kinds of practices that bring with them pleasure,

tradition, history, culture, etc.). Whether we find the meal in a pill hor-
rifying or liberating, it is clear that functional foods, as central features
of our diet, seem increasingly inevitable and increasingly omnipresent on
our grocery store shelves. These kinds of foods may not have always been
inevitable, but they have become part of our common sense view of food
because of a series of political, social, economic, technological, and linguistic
choices that helped the ideology of nutritionism prosper and advance. The
building of an artificial world through chemistry could prevent starvation
and improve public health, or so the food futurists thought. But what is
at stake in the pursuit of this kind of future?

As we move closer to the meal in a pill we also seem to find increasing amounts of evidence of diet-related diseases. Perhaps the meal in the
pill could solve such public health issues, but it is more likely the case
that the entire ideology of nutritionism has had a hand in the invention
of the evidence for the ill effects of a bad diet. I am not denying the
existence of a link between diet and disease, but this link points to the
manner in which the very concept of health is figured within the science of
nutrition. A discourse of quantification makes possible a notion of health
as the absence of disease not as a state of complete well-being. If there
is a link between diet and disease, then we all have the ability to fend
off potential sickness by eating correctly. But if we follow the regimens
offered by the USDA what will we be able to say about the state of our
well-being? Does the evidence of diet-related disease really leave us with an
adequate conception of health and well-being if that conception is devoid
of pleasure, tradition, taste, and so forth? A complete answer to those
questions may not be possible, but at the very least denaturalizing the
ideology of nutritionism should help us reflect on, and critically examine,
claims about the relationship between diet and disease by pointing to the
deeper conception of health at stake within discourses of quantification.

The future of eating, farming practices, the environment, global
economies, public health, history, memory, tradition, and pleasure are all
at stake in the story of the quantification of food. The manner in which
we typically understand food and eating, in other words our common
sense approach to the question of what we should eat, is a product of a
controlling ideology of nutritionism. This ideology is founded on practices
of quantification. Those practices have sought to eliminate vocabularies of
pleasure, taste, and tradition in the name of public health. But we must
ask whether we are willing to sacrifice these other possible futures for
a meal in a pill. If we continue to eat foods because of their nutritional
portfolio, will we miss some other aspects of eating that are equally as
valuable? And will we really improve our own health in so doing? The

evidence seems to suggest that such eating practices do not, in fact, improve public health, yet we continue to pursue the ideology of nutritionism with ever-greater zeal. As critical history, I hope that this book serves as reason to pause and ponder whether or not our common sense view of food and eating is really worth holding onto, or whether that view is likely to produce a future of food devoid of what matters most. Health, after all, can mean much more than being free from illness.

Chapter One

The Early History of American Nutrition Research

From Quality to Quantity

On May 15, 1862, President Abraham Lincoln approved a bill to establish the United States Department of Agriculture. The USDA was born with $60,000 in six rooms in the basement of the Patent Office building.[1] Drawing from the European import of a scientific approach to agriculture, which relied largely on the nascent field of chemistry, the USDA's directive was to advance scientific research. The department was "laying the foundation for becoming a great science-producing agency of government" (Cochrane, 1993, p. 96). It was the expressed goal of the newfound department to: "Test by experiment the use of agricultural implements and the value of seeds, soils, manures, and animals; undertake the chemical investigation of soils, grains, fruits, vegetables, and manures, publishing the results."[2] From cotton to cattle to cucumbers, the USDA had an array of directions in which to take their scientific research.

In the years after the approval of this bill, federally funded scientists, in USDA-sanctioned labs, set to unearthing the chemical components of food, and the physiological processes of digestion. Chemists used the process of calorimetry to break food down into calories, fats, proteins, and carbohydrates. Techniques of dehydration, precipitation, and combustion reduced foods to their constituent molecular parts. These experiments, as well as experiments using the calorimeter to quantify human action, rendered the relationship between food and eater measurable. The emerging science of nutrition introduced the notion of the balanced human-food equation based on the zero-waste model of the combustion engine. In order for maximum efficiency in the human body, the input of food must equal the output of work. The USDA thought that understanding these two quantities, the calories in food and the calories used by metabolism, could improve the lives of Americans.

While chemical catabolism occurred in the laboratory, creating new knowledge about food, the laboratory lexicon served as the new language to discuss it. The terms of science were old, but their application to food was new. In these early experiments, a scientific language was mobilized to make food a quantifiable entity. A cool, creamy glass of milk became 150 calories and a measurable ratio of fat, proteins, and carbohydrates. The scientific and systematic analysis of foods by the USDA created both knowledge about food and a method for its communication. The scientific treatment of food, the categorization and charting of the constituent nutrients of everything edible, and the grading of food on its proportions of these quantifiable components mark an important moment in the development of American nutrition.

This chapter lays the historical groundwork for how a language of quantification became the preferred mode of communication in federal food policy, and it outlines the United States Department of Agriculture's early use of numbers, measures, and standards. Such a historical foundation demonstrates the coproduction of scientific knowledge and a numeric language of food. From the birth of the USDA in 1862, its implementation of science as the disciplinary framework of knowledge production determined the type of information the agency produced. By default, science provided the language with which to produce new knowledge about domestic agriculture. Because food fell under the aegis of the department, the government body's advice on food and "good" or "proper" eating (the former being under its jurisdiction and the latter implicated in the former) has never extended its discursive reach beyond the language of science, scientific methods, and the cornerstones of this discipline: numbers, measures, and quantitative comparison. The late 19th- and early 20th-century agriculture laboratories, through their research mandates, publications, and formation of a scientific community, gave birth to and encouraged the proliferation of a discourse of quantification.

Within this newfound science of food, new technologies were in place to produce knowledge and encourage the use of a discourse steeped in numbers and calculations. The chemical and calorimetric analysis of foods using the technologies that produced numeric data perpetuated a language of quantification and measures that allowed for, and encouraged, normalization, standardization, and objectification of qualitative judgments about taste. The language of numbers and standards allowed for the objective comparison of apples to oranges to steak to sugar. Therefore, I use this history to argue that early federal scientific and quantitative communication of food conflated the idea of *quality* with the idea of *quantity*. *How much* of something became the marker for *how good* it was. Thus, *quality* food was determined by *quantitative* terms.

Federal Agricultural Science:
The Mandate of the USDA and the Hatch Act

In 1862, the same year Lincoln founded the U.S. Department of Agriculture, increased contact between American and European scientists created a growing interest in improving agricultural practices (Gates, 1965, p. 255). In his first annual report the commissioner of the USDA, appropriately named Isaac Newton, declared that

> It shall be the duty of the Board to watch the interests of agriculture as they are or may be affected by the legislation of the country; to make such reports, memorials and recommendations, as may advance the cause of agriculture, promote and diffuse agricultural knowledge . . . and to show the importance of science to agriculture. (Qtd. in True, 1937, p. 37)

These reports would become the gold standard for work at the USDA, and they are still, today, one of the central markers of the scientific ethos intrinsically tied to this branch of the government.

A chemist published the first scientific paper in the department. The paper was a report on the chemical analysis of grapes wherein American chemists concluded that domestic grapes were as good as any European grapes for making wine. Obviously, French vintners would find such a conclusion amusing and dead wrong. But by reducing grapes to their chemical constituents such an argument becomes possible. Reports and papers followed on sugar beets and the chemistry of sugar manufacturing, stone fruits, sweet potatoes, peanuts, edible fungi, tea and coffee substitutes, butter and edible oils, baking powders, and meat extracts. In 1869 a staff chemist called attention to the excessive adulteration of foodstuffs and the need to maintain and monitor the purity of these products by chemical means.[3] These early papers hinted at the extent to which the scientists at the USDA would be involved in federal policy and public communication. In *Science in the Federal Government*, American political historian Hunter Dupree (1957) states that these acts of 1862 "mark a genuine turning point for science in the government" (p. 149). Prior to 1862 scientific institutions lacked constitutional status, largely due to internal incoherence and conflict between institutions. With governmental support and structure, science and agriculture were given a political space in which to proliferate.

While the creation of the USDA marked the government's commitment to federal scientific research in agriculture, the Morrill Land Grant College Act, passed in the same year as the formation of the USDA, aided scientists who needed laboratory space to perform their experiments. The Land Grant College Act did not affiliate the laboratories with the federal government or the USDA, but the act endowed the individual states with public land to be sold, the profits of which were used as financial boosters to colleges of agriculture.[4] Within the agricultural colleges, the act's money created state experiment stations. These stations provided laboratory space and research facilities to those studying the scientific applications of agriculture. But the Land Grant College Act provided more than a physical space for scientists. Because chemistry and botany were the only mature disciplines assumed by the new stations, "agriculture" itself was not yet defined. The physical space of the laboratory was influential in establishing the field of agriculture, and the kind of work in which the scientists were to engage. The experiment stations encouraged the professional self-definition of agricultural *science*, and the Land Grant College Act abetted the creation of a new scientific discipline (Danbom, 1986).

At the Convention of the Association of American Agricultural Colleges and Experiment Stations, speaker M. H. Buckam posited that the Land Grant College Act had brought "the light of learning and the aid of science to bear upon those pursuits and callings which . . . would thus be lifted to the plane of the other professions and confer equal respectability upon their members."[5] Science had social value, and it imported structure and respect to agriculture. Experiment station scientists performed the agricultural experiments that the individual farmer (who lacked time, opportunity, and often a formal education) could not.[6] The transposition of experimental science upon agriculture elevated farming and made it a profession requiring special knowledge and skill. Instead of agricultural knowledge creation in the hands of the "hicks, yokels and ignorant bumpkins," whose approach to agriculture relied on intuition and experience, the newfound scientific and quantitative approach put agriculture into terms that were bound, concrete, well defined, comparable, and verifiable (Rosenberg, 1977, p. 403). This national effort to encourage a rational approach to agriculture served to redefine the terms of agriculture itself. The experiment station scientist was encouraged by what Charles Rosenberg calls "the ideological primacy of science and agriculture" to commit to a set of professional values that influenced American science at this time (1976, pp. 171–172). Encouraged by the institutions to stimulate economic development and interest in pure science, the experiment station scientists were empowered to establish the language of communication for this new marriage of the farm and hard facts.

The first experiment station in the United States was in Connecticut. This station was established by the efforts of Yale professor Samuel Johnson and his former student, Wilbur Olin Atwater. The two men were active promoters of agricultural research in the United States, and Johnson had served as the advisor to President Lincoln when the creation of the USDA was signed into law. Johnson and Atwater were largely responsible for the establishment of the experiment stations' scientific credo. In later years, the USDA credited Atwater with showing the experiment station to be "primarily and fundamentally a scientific institution" that "undoubtedly had a broad influence in the further development of such institutions in the United States" (True, 1937, p. 85). The Connecticut Experiment Station in Storrs, affiliated with Wesleyan University, specialized in chemical analyses of fertilizers and foods. Johnson and Atwater were both European-trained chemists who had worked in German agricultural chemistry laboratories that specialized in nutritional chemistry. Johnson's German mentor and pioneer of the nutritional sciences, Justus von Liebig, largely influenced the direction of his research, and the methods he used in the Connecticut experiment station. Americans and Europeans alike considered Liebig the founder of experimental agricultural and nutrition sciences. He trained scientists from all over the world in his lab in Giessen and specialized in eudiometric analyses of organic elements in foods.[7]

Liebig developed a distinctly quantitative approach to nutrition from his studies in inorganic chemistry, in which he used highly efficient and precise techniques of chemical analysis. In the 1830s he used those techniques to begin studying the chemical processes of living organisms. He first studied plants and the chemical constitution of soil, water, and air. This led him to the conclusion that the nutrient substances of plants were inorganic, rather than organic. From this insight he was able to invent artificial fertilizers. Therefore, Liebig's move into the chemical analysis of plants opened up new and important connections between chemistry and industry because he could promise greater productivity of food. He used this same emphasis on improved productivity in his work on animal chemistry. In 1842 he published *Animal Chemistry*, in which he claimed that "the only method which can lead to their [animals] final resolution, namely, the *quantitative* method, has been employed" (Liebig, 1842, p. xxii). Liebig's approach was to measure and analyze the foods taken in by the animal, and the products that were exhaled or excreted. On the basis of such analyses, he proposed a great deal of theoretical speculation about the chemical processes of the body. Thus animal and human nutrition depended on chemical changes that could be assessed by the calculation of the relation of inputs and outputs.[8] The point of this approach was to assess, quantitatively, the relationship between what was consumed as food and what was expended as work and heat in both the animal and human body. This concern with work and physical efficiency became a central preoccupation of early American nutrition research.

The Storrs experiment station research reflected Johnson's European training under Liebig. Starting around 1880, the American chemists used a modified Bertholet bomb calorimeter to begin determining the heats of combustion of a variety of foods. The Bertholet bomb calorimeter was considered to be the perfect technique for determining the heat and energy equivalents of carbon-containing compounds and built upon Atwater and Johnson's eudiometric nitrogen research under Liebig. The Connecticut research station began producing and publishing studies of the chemical composition of foods and became known as the station concerned with the nutrition of man and animals (True, 1937, p. 153).

Samuel Johnson and Wilber Atwater were highly prized consultants to the USDA due largely to their experiences in government-funded European experiment stations. The two men gave direction and advice to the government and became vocal promoters for the establishment of federally regulated and funded agricultural research. American scientists returning from European labs came back with technical knowledge and a new vision of how science ought to be pursued, and what contributions it could make to the American public (Ashby, 1959). In USDA publications, Atwater began writing in favor of adopting the European model of the scientific laboratory in domestic experiment stations.[9] From 1885 to 1887 Johnson and Atwater served as agricultural science advisors to Congress and made the push for support of federal appropriations for the experiment stations. After lengthy debate, President Grover Cleveland signed the Hatch Experiment Station Act on March 2, 1887. This act changed the financial structure of the experiment stations and formed an alliance between the USDA and the heretofore independent experiment stations. Prior to the passage of the Hatch Act, the Department of Agriculture found it difficult to coordinate and keep track of what was going on at each station. This new alliance (and allotment of funds) allowed the government to standardize and influence what the research scientists in each station should be doing and how they should be doing it.

The Hatch Act was a nationwide subsidization of research in agriculture by the federal government. After the act passed, the state experiment stations became the joint responsibility of both the federal and state governments, and the stations developed a formal relationship with the USDA. Each state received an annual federal grant of $15,000 to maintain their experiment station if they had one. In addition to the financial handout, the Hatch Act provided a structure and mandate that directed and defined the activities of the experiment stations and their scientists. The act stated that the goal of experiment stations was:

To acquire and diffuse among the people of the United States, useful and practical information . . . and that it should be the object and duty of said experiment stations to conduct original researches [sic] or verify experiments on the physiology of plants and animals.[10]

Federally controlled experiment stations were enormously successful in Europe, and the European-trained American scientists felt that with more attention paid to agricultural science, the United States could surpass Europe in the advancement of agricultural science.[11] The Hatch Act was seen as the best way in which applications of science could "increase [agricultural] production at a decreased cost" and promote the precision of scientific methods that had come to define the USDA as the "foremost agency for the advancement of agricultural science" (True, 1937, p. 126).

Through the establishment of the USDA and the passage of the Morrill Land Grant College Act and the Hatch Act, the American government demonstrated its scientific directive. The promotion of science and the federal sanctions now circumscribing agriculture came to constitute the mission of the USDA. These acts also bestowed upon federal scientists the institutional values of a scientific ethos. The federal mandate of science enabled its normative structure to take root and thus demarcate patterns of knowledge production. These acts established the experiment stations as centers of knowledge production, and the experiment station scientists as knowledge producers. As Robert Merton (1974) notes, the institutional values of science that are "transmitted by precept and example and reinforced by sanctions . . . in varying degrees internalized by the scientist, thus fashioning his scientific conscience," became the foundation for agricultural knowledge production in America (p. 269). By adopting and encouraging science as epistemological bedrock, certain kinds of knowledge, kinds that could be, according to Merton, "empirically confirmed" and "logically consistent," were the prized products of the newly defined discipline of agriculture (p. 270). Agriculture, its practices, and its discourse became shaped by the professional standards of the scientist.

In 1888, the year following the passage of the Hatch Act, the government noted some "irregularities" in the use of the federal funds by some of the states. In order to abate inappropriate use of funds, the USDA created the Office of Experiment Stations, a federal sentinel for the activities of the stations. The government gave the Office of Experiment Stations, or OES, the power to regularly monitor and appraise the research projects financed by government money. The OES, entirely run by European-trained American scientists, sought a European model for the stations and their experiments: clearly delineated research that used verifiable scientific principles, uninfluenced by bureaucratic impulses or political interference. The stations were not to be purveyors of general information on agriculture; they were autonomous, science-serving institutions (Harding, 1947; Ferleger, 1990a).

To generate scientific spirit among the experiment station scientists and to provide a standard for written communication among them, the OES published the *Experiment Station Record*. An important source of information, the *ESR* was a collection of scientific papers from Hatch Act–established American agricultural experiment stations and abroad. The OES made it known that the *ESR* was not a forum for swapping farm practices or tricks of the farming trade. The *ESR* published scientific abstracts, experiment results, papers, and both domestic and foreign agricultural science news. Stations were heavily criticized by the OES if they merely presented well-known farm practices to popular audiences. Often times the experiment station scientists felt bound by their instructional duties at the land grant colleges and lectured or wrote at the undergraduate level instead of at the level of the chemist or agronomist. Furthermore, the stations were chastised for being mere "bureaus of information or education" and warned that resources that were depleted during these activities would not be recuperated. Any activities that experiment station scientists engaged in should not detract from their scientific inquiries. This mandate ensured that experiment station scientists, though they may not all write or communicate using scientific conventions, could read them in the *ESR*.

The Hatch Act also mandated that each experiment station or affiliated college report its research to the USDA and publish its experiments in quarterly experiment station bulletins (which contained only the research of the individual experiment station) and the national *Experiment Station Record*. In addition to keeping scientists abreast of national experiment station laboratory work, the *ESR* held the scientists accountable to particular standards of research and the appropriate communication of that research. Knowing that their research was going to be nationally circulated among fellow scientists ensured the upholding of, and attention to, scientific detail and the attendance to scientific language—acts of public communication could supposedly insure the precision and value of experiments.

The *Record* provided scientists with a disciplinary framework that could guide their style of communication. Experiment reports contained lists of apparatuses, methods of experimentation, and numeric data. In addition to developing a cohesive scientific standard for written discourse among the scientists, the USDA recommended that the experiment stations form regional or national associations or affiliate themselves with the Association of Official Agricultural Chemistry or Society for the Promotion of Agricultural Science. These associations provided scientists with behavioral guidelines for the profession, and helped shape the research initiatives of the scientists and provided ideas for "intelligent lines of inquiry" (True, 1937, pp. 119–120).

By acting as a clearinghouse for the laboratory experiment reports, and by encouraging association among scientists, the OES and the *Experiment Station Record* strengthened the USDA's commitment to the marriage of science and agriculture and perpetuated and inculcated the structures and language of science, the rigidity of experimentation and method, and the need for objective and quantifiable results. The *ESR* represented a palpable instantiation of the attitude of the new science of agriculture. By encouraging the scientific form and style of agricultural knowledge, the *ESR* restricted access to new agricultural information to those who could speak the language of science. According to Scott Montgomery (1996), "such inaccessibility alone has the power to intimidate" and allows for the occlusion of lay language, and by extension, lay knowledge (pp. 7–8). This application of the language of science to the ordinary farming routine, served to shift the persona of the agricultural expert from the farmer, who was scientifically illiterate, to the USDA chemists, botanists, and veterinarians. The process of the nomination of practices by science, practices that were once accessible to the laity, rendered them scientific phenomena, to be explored only by those who could manage this new language.

When the Office of Experiment Stations came into existence, Wilbur Atwater became its director. While the immediate function of the OES was to regulate and coordinate experiment station work, it also sought to point research in what it deemed to be scientifically fruitful and socially useful directions. The Hatch Act clause calling for the diffusion of "useful and practical information" was subject to various interpretations. The USDA's commitment to science did not define public lectures to farmers as useful and practical. The Office of Experiment Stations acted as a scientific watchdog that ensured that the experiment station expenditures were made in accordance with the spirit of the Hatch Act. Atwater was encouraged to "secure, as far as practicable, uniformity of methods and results in the word of [experiment] stations and to furnish forms, as far as practicable, for the tabulation of results, of investigations or experiments."[12]

The nomination of Atwater to the position of OES director was central to the ideological shift that was taking place in the USDA in the late 19th century. While almanac-type knowledge was quaint and perhaps useful to some, Atwater insisted that agricultural experiment stations needed more scientific agriculture and laboratory research. "Abstract" research that specialized in verifiable scientific particulars, was preferred to the approach of the holistic farming "system."[13] The designation of the "professional" scientist at the helm of agricultural knowledge production fit neatly into the zeitgeist of the American population at that time, who equated moral efficiency and social order with professionalization and bureaucratization (Haskell, 2000; Wiebe, 1967). The rhetorical force of the formally educated scientist easily displaced the simple and provincial farmer as the voice of agricultural authority (Haskell, 1984, pp. 28–83).

In *American Science in the Age of Jackson*, George Daniels (1968) writes that the abstraction of a "body of knowledge from the public domain is a necessary first step in creating a place for a society of experts. . . . It is incumbent upon the profession to demonstrate that it is in the interest of society at large to support a special group in the cultivation of esoteric knowledge" (p. 41). Because the USDA supported their research, the experiment station scientist was supported by the "public" to produce knowledge. As the government used science as new rhetorical muscle and claimed that it was to be performed in a certain way, by accredited people, in particular places, to produce "special knowledge," other discourses of agriculture and, by extension, food, became of fringe value to the federal government. At the USDA, the shift from lay knowledge to the socially influential professional knowledge augmented and perpetuated the institution's default manner of communication. Science was the mother tongue of federal agriculture and scientists were the native speakers. This fluency afforded the federal experiment station scientist the social authority to advance the application of this style of communication to all agricultural matters from fertilizers to butter adulteration to the fecundity of Guernsey cows.

Wilbur Olin Atwater, "der Vater of American Nutrition"

The director of the Office of Experiment Stations, Wilbur Atwater, was the chemist and principal scientist at the Connecticut Experiment Station at Wesleyan University. Atwater had received his PhD in 1869 from Yale University under Samuel Johnson, and then completed a postdoctoral course of study in Europe at the universities of Leipzig and Berlin. There, Atwater saw the workings of the German experiment station, which provided him with an archetype for nascent American agricultural science. Atwater's European experiences in the laboratories of German chemists and physiologists further focused his academic interests on the interactions and applications of agriculture and human nutrition. Importing the European model of nutrition research and the experiment station was vital to the construction of the discourse and knowledge of the science of nutrition as it emerged in America. Atwater's position at the OES allowed him to push the agricultural experiment station research toward a more scientific and experiment based approach. While assuming the position of director of experiment stations, Atwater maintained his post as the director of the Connecticut Experiment Station at Wesleyan to pursue his own research interests. Atwater was an outspoken advocate for the federally funded research lab and after the passage of the Hatch Act and his appointment as the office director, many of the stations feared that Atwater's position at the office might influence the allocation of any additional research funds. Atwater resigned as director of the office in 1891 to pursue his research at the Connecticut Experiment Station. While Atwater's resignation removed him from appearing to directly influence congressional appropriation of funds for specific agricultural research projects, he received the first appropriation in 1894, allocated to his laboratory for research on human nutrition.

Atwater's doctoral dissertation, "The Proximate Composition of Several Types of American Maize," represented the first series of food analyses by modern methods in the United States. At Wesleyan, the U.S. commissioner of fisheries funded Atwater to analyze the different species of fish eaten in the United States, and Atwater used the method of proximate analysis to do so. Proximate analysis entailed determining the crude protein, fat and carbohydrate ratios of foodstuffs. While the method served the purpose of producing quantitative determinations of food components, the imprecision of the technique frustrated Atwater. Because the analysis had to be performed in the open air, impurities, residual moisture, and loss of extractable materials made it difficult to obtain reproducible results (Atwater, 1878).

In 1882–1883, Atwater received a federal grant to study whether humans could digest fish as well as they could meat, and he headed to Germany to begin the study. At the University of Munich, he worked in the laboratory of Carl von Voit, protégé of Justus von Liebig. Voit, a leading nutritional chemist, was fascinated with human metabolism and the physical and chemical principles of human intake and output. With his cadre of chemists, Voit explored the idea that proteins, fats, and carbohydrates all had different effects on the body because they stimulated the body's metabolic processes at different rates. Voit concluded that the mass and capacity of human cells determine the total metabolism. The human "machine" Voit found, worked best when it had sufficient calories to fuel the engine (in the form of fats and carbohydrates) and sufficient protein to restore and retain muscular tissue. The ideas of Voit and his colleague Max Rubner facilitated the application of reductionist, determinist, and positivist ideas to the interaction between humans and their food. A central issue in 19th-century German science was the determination of the chemical composition of food, and the best foods to eat in order to maximize human output (Cravens, 1996).[14] Voit's lab gave Atwater his first taste of the European procedures for studying human nutrition, and the attempts that the Munich group were making to put social and economic values on foods based on their contributions of protein and energy to the human body (Carpenter, 1986).

While Voit's studies were inconclusive, and later bettered by Rubner, his interest in *stoffwechsel*, or the chemical theory of metabolic substances, was vital to the then-popular concept of the body as a de-animated machine. Voit's theory of the metabolization of food treated the body as a Helmholtzian motor, whose non-energetic needs could be ignored (Rabinbach, 1990). This model of the human motor allowed for the concurrent birth of a discourse of quantification of foodstuffs, as well as the quantification of human activity. While the *stoffwechsel* framework was too rudimentary to develop a complete theory of human motor-food interaction, Voit's casting of the Helmholtz-human brought together and solidified the concept of enumerated food and quantifiable human activity. If Voit could accurately count food, and food fueled humans, then it would not be long before technological innovation could allow for the determination of the waste-free balance between human food intake and physical output.

Voit's goal of determining the human *kraftwechsel*, "a mathematically reliable system of equivalence between the amount of potential energy ingested in the form of nutriments and the amount of energy produced" (Rabinbach, 1990, p. 126) remained out of his reach until the development of the room calorimeter. But it was in Voit's lab that Atwater first worked with a government-funded human respiration calorimeter. This precursor to the room calorimeter was the fundamental tool in testing the laws of human energetics, the application of the first law of thermodynamics to the human body, and in creating quantitative distinctions between foods and their interaction in the human body. Food taken into the body was transformed through digestion into a set of discrete metabolites that could be extrapolated through the human output of gas. Calorimetry made Atwater's technique of proximate analysis seem simple and imprecise. But the European technology of calorimetry furnished Atwater with an enumerated discourse to apply to food: a language of caloric quantities. Atwater's experience with the German calorimeter gave insight into the future of technologies of nutritional science, as well as a rhetoric in which to express the results of the technology, which fit into the already established framework of scientific communication encouraged by the USDA.

The calorimeter was a cornerstone technology for the application of science to human food, to the organization of new knowledge about food, and to the integration of numeric language for communication about food. In other words, the creation of the American notion of nutrition, or the science of food, relied on the federal government's embrace of the scientific method to further agriculture, as well as the import of scientific technologies and ideas about food and the human body. The technology of the calorimeter availed a language of numbers to the discursive community of scientists already in place at the USDA, and acted to set the agenda for nutrition research to follow. A technology of quantification like the calorimeter was "simultaneously a means of planning and of prediction" (Porter, 1995, p. 43). This newfound ability to measure food forged a numeric relationship between food and human activity and provided a set of scientifically appropriate terms to define that relationship. Thus, calorimetric measurements were not demonstrating a theory, but they were manifestations of a technology that could be used in future to manage human activity and structure and give meaning to scientific practice.

Human Calorimetry: The Technology of Nutrition

In late 1886, just prior to the passage of the Hatch Act, Atwater returned to Germany, this time to the laboratory of Max Rubner. Rubner, a laboratory colleague of Atwater's from Voit's lab, had modified the Voit calorimeter and began to study the heat energy equivalence of foodstuffs. Rubner had established his own laboratory and began investigating the human body in a new way with a new calorimetric tool: the room calorimeter. Rubner's interest was in the science of energetics. He believed that calories were the human fuel, and he conceived the body as a combustion engine. This parallel allowed Rubner to extend the first law of thermodynamics, the law of conservation of energy, to people. The room calorimeter fit Rubner's concept of the closed system body/machine, in which he could ensure that the total energy of the system remained constant. Rubner had people enter the room calorimeter and perform a variety of tasks for which he measured the output of respiration gases. With this apparatus, Rubner could determine more than just the number of calories in a food, the limitation of bomb calorimetry. Now he could determine how many calories of *human* energy foods yielded. Rubner discovered that when fueled by fats, the human body gleaned twice as much caloric energy as when fueled by sugars or proteins.

The room calorimeter became the ultimate arbiter of the quantification of human activity and established a numeric relationship between food intake and physical output. It could measure the calories going into the human, and the calories going out for any given (albeit room-restricted) activity. Together with determining how much energy the human machine expended, Rubner collected caloric data and chemical analyses of commonly consumed foods. The data of energy expenditure, along with the data of energy available in food, gave birth to a simple human mathematical equation.[15] Calorimetry could determine how much you should put into your body, based on how much you put out.

Human calorimetry impressed Atwater. In it he saw a leveling, rational, and impartial approach to food with myriad applications to ameliorate American society. The USDA had experimented with food, and Atwater himself was very fond of determining nutrient ratios of foods through combustion, but nutritional experimentation on the interaction of food and humans was uncharted waters. The deficiency of domestic nutritional technology, one that had so much scientific, social, and economic potential, frustrated Atwater, and he became more vocal and insistent that it was in America's best interest to perform calorimetric analyses of American food in conjunction with tests of human digestibility and fuel value. Atwater became a vocal and prolific advocate of the benefits of the application of science to food, and he began to write about food, the American diet, and the importance of good nutrition in USDA publications as well as in the public press.[15] In 1887 he wrote a series of articles entitled "The Chemistry of Food and Nutrition" for *Century Magazine*, a magazine that circulated widely among the middle-class public. In this publication, Atwater outlined America's problems with its diet: overconsumption of sweets, wasteful spending on expensive cuts of meat, and too little attention to the diet in general. He called for the public to better themselves through education in the science of nutrition:

> Among those who desire to economize there is great pecuniary loss from the selection of materials in which the nutrients are really, though not apparently, dearer than need be. . . . Our task is to learn how our food builds up our bodies, repairs their wastes, yields heat and energy, and how we may select and use our food-materials to the best advantage of health and purse. (Atwater, 1887b, pp. 59–60)

Atwater encouraged education in nutritional science but apologized to the readers of *Century Magazine* for his abstract scientific explanations: "[I should] make these articles not too abstrusely scientific and avoid the tone and language of the college lecture-room as [they] are unsuited to the pages of a magazine. But I must crave a little latitude; the results of scientific research cannot be explained without some tedious technicalities and dry details" (p. 60). Thus the article proceeded to outline, in detail, the process of bomb calorimetry (including apparatus diagrams), the importance of the chemical analyses of foods' fats, protein and carbohydrate contents (including a chart of the percentages of the contents for 70 foods), and the chemical and mineral composition of the human body. At several points, Atwater waxes about the superiority of the American worker to the European, the superiority of the domestic soil in producing nutritionally rich foods, and the productivity of the American workforce. Despite these advantages, Atwater was embittered by the fact that America still lacked a human calorimeter:

In the German laboratories, particularly, one finds not only the needed apparatus, but what is no less important, trained assistants and servants. [Why must we] seek the fundamental data of our [food] studies in the learned and profound research of foreign universities? (p. 73)

Atwater's push for the passage of the Hatch Act was spurred largely by his desire for an American calorimeter in his own Wesleyan experiment station.

His Connecticut laboratory was a successful institution for nutritional agricultural research, and the Hatch Act allowed Atwater to pursue his goal of emulating the European laboratory experience, where federal funds were availed to perform large-scale scientific work. Determining the chemical composition of foods was important, but it was at the level of human interaction with food via calorimetry that nutrition work represented practical social value. Atwater saw the calorimeter as a social liberator: Americans who understood the science of nutrition could be healthier, save money, and live happier lives. If Americans understood food in terms of quantities: calories, percentages, and rations, they could determine their daily nutritional needs and eat accordingly. With enough scientific research into the workings of food and its interaction with the human body, nutrition could save the health and wealth of American citizens.

With Atwater as the numerate emissary of the calorie, the push began to fund wide-scale research into American nutrition and a domestic calorimeter. The USDA could easily justify an apparatus whose data could ameliorate American society. In 1893 an *Office of Experiment Stations Bulletin* printed an article entitled "Suggestions for the Establishment of Food Laboratories in Connection with the Agricultural Experiment Stations of the United States," wherein the authors made the plea for an allotment of federal money that was "a small additional appropriation in order to complete the service and to round out the whole science of nutrition by including the nutrition of mankind as a final object of the whole work" (Atwater, 1893). Because nutrition was such a worthwhile course of study, and because it had far-reaching benefits, this money was to be separate from, and in addition to, the Hatch Act funds.

In the first yearbook of the USDA in 1894, Atwater authored the article "Food and Diet." This article contained charts, classifications, and lists of food. In this article, he wrote about food's relative nutritive value to the body, and economic value to the family, while emphasizing the importance of knowledge of nutrition, and his own dietary research:

> With the progress of human knowledge and human experience we are at last coming to see that the human body needs the closest care . . . and that among the things essential to health and wealth, to right thinking and right living, is our diet. (p. 357)

Atwater concludes with a plea for support for more research:

> [W]hat is now most needed is research. Of the fundamental laws of nutrition we know as yet too little. Of the actual practice of people and their food economy, our knowledge is equally deficient. More thorough study of the research of man is very much needed. (p. 359)

For the fiscal year of 1895, Congress made an appropriation of $10,000 for investigations on the nutritive value of human foods, with "a view to determining ways in which the dietaries [*sic*] of our people might be made more wholesome and more economical" (p. 387).[17] This project was carried on in conjunction with the state colleges and experiment stations with Atwater as the special agent in charge of the investigations.

Atwater used a portion of the government money allotted to human nutrition research to complete, in 1897, the first U.S. human respiration calorimeter based largely on the calorimeter design of Voit and Rubner. With the help of Wesleyan physicist E. B. Rosa, Atwater perfected a respiration calorimeter that produced results of enviable accuracy. The calorimeter was a large copper-lined wooden box about 170 cubic feet, large enough to accommodate a folding bed or table, or whatever athletic apparatus the experiment required. What was most amazing about the calorimeter, aside from the fact that it worked, was that the subjects appeared to remain reasonably well and comfortable during their calorimetric incarceration that lasted, on average, four or five nights. Along with resting and active metabolic rates, Atwater tested for brain energy expenditure by having college students take their examinations in the calorimeter.

This newfound technology revealed precise measurements about human energy expenditure. By monitoring the change in temperature in the room during the human subject's various activities, the calorimeter determined the quantities of nutrients and energy that the human subject metabolized during different physical activities. It established the relationship between expended energy and metabolized energy, as well as the digestion and assimilation of foods. The Atwater-Rosa calorimeter could recover 99.8% of the carbon dioxide expelled by the subject during the experiment and 99.9% of the heat produced by the human subject, as well as the substrates they metabolized. The system allowed for the measure of the balance between food intake and energy output and the quantification of the dynamics of human digestion. The Atwater-Rosa calorimeter gave the calorie human implications. In order to determine human metabolism calculations, Atwater used his new technology in conjunction with a bomb calorimeter. The bomb calorimeter allowed Atwater to burn foods to determine their energy values as well as burning the excreted products of the room calorimeter's human subject. Used together, both apparatuses could measure the body's energy expenditure as the difference between the food input and human "output" (Wiggen, 1993). The room calorimeter was capable of amazingly precise measurements of human metabolism. It could record a change in room temperature if the human subject so much as wound her watch.

Prior to the merge of the data of the bomb and respiration calorimeters, food's numeric information was external to the food itself. A food's quantities dealt strictly with extrinsic amounts, numbers that could be determined through gross weights and measures. The quantities of fats, protein, and sugars in a foodstuff when they were burned and weighed in a laboratory oven were important information. But by studying the digestibility and metabolization of foods, Atwater determined that in the human body fat yields 9 calories of energy per gram, and carbohydrates and proteins each 4 calories per gram. These Atwater units of metabolizable energy of foods based on the chemical composition were the linchpins in the study of American nutrition.[18]

Wilbur Atwater's process of experimentation and innovation to perpetuate the "calorification" of food could be compared with Robert

Millikan's determination of the charge on the electron. As outlined by Ian Hacking (1983), experiments that establish *constants*, or numeric values that change in no appreciable way over time, confer epistemic clout to those who pioneer the experiment (p. 236). In the case of Atwater and his determination of the Atwater units, his innovation of the extraordinarily accurate calorimeter enshrined the quantitative model of food and eating, because there were always new numbers and knowledge to produce, and no challenge to their verity. The numeric regularity of Atwater's work established these ratios, as Hacking puts it, as constants that "transfer mathematical use to the description of the world." The surety of the constants, the "positivist regularities," is "the intended harvest of science" (pp. 61–63). Just as the calorimeter became the terra firma technology for producing scientific and numeric knowledge about food, the establishment of the Atwater units fortified the foundation upon which nutrition could become *the* framework for understanding food, and numbers its qualitative adjectives. Hacking (1990) writes: "The numbers are called fundamental because they occur as parameters in the fundamental laws of nature. Such a picture is implicitly hierarchical. First come the laws, then the constants that fix their parameters, and then a set of boundary conditions" (p. 56). And so, the calorimeter became the instrument for knowledge production, and Atwater the namesake to the numeric knowledge the instrument produced. The Atwater units then, became the language of the calorimeter.

For every food that the calorimeter burned, the instrument spoke to the scientist through its heat readings and ash analysis. The idea was that the calorimeter could communicate information about things like motion or protein content and establish it as natural fact. In *Instruments and the Imagination*, Hankins and Silverman (1995) make a similar point. They argue that instruments, such as the calorimeter, are "things whose purpose it is to help us analyze and reason about other things. They are things that we construct to represent and interpret nature" (p. 9). Through facilitating analysis and reason, and by communicating and representing knowledge through quantitative readings, the calorimeter produced words imbued with scientific meaning:

> Words were more than arbitrary symbols for things; they con-
> tained hidden signification, so that through one word one could
> learn about the thing. It was a kind of secret language that
> signified more than the images and words taken by themselves
> could mean. It was also secret in the sense that only those
> learned individuals who had been initiated into the meaning
> of those images and words could understand it. (p. 8)

The calorimeter was a fundamental tool in shaping and organizing a discourse of quantification and the science of nutrition. Because "reading" the calorimeter required one to speak the "secret language," the scientist became the interpreter between the calorimeter and the ideas it produced. As with many scientific instruments, the calorimeter "determined what is possible, and what is possible determines to a large extent, what can be thought" (p. 5).

Through his research with the two calorimeters, Atwater determined how many calories foods yielded in the human body. Once a term used exclusively in the laboratory of physical chemists and physicists, with its application to human nutrition, *calorie* had now taken on a new meaning. Human calorimetry experiments transformed the calorie from a unit of physical science, to a unit of human fodder, and finally, through Atwater's application, a determinant of quality.[19] The calorie made food something outside of just eating and the sensation of taste. Food became something to calculate, measure, and empirically "know." The application of the once solely scientific calorie to the human diet represents a pivotal moment in the establishment of an American epistemology of food and eating. When federal agricultural science adopted the structures and means of empirical research, the calorie became an integral part of the lexicon of human nourishment.

Normalizing the Eater and Rationalizing Quality

In 1896, Atwater published "The Chemical Composition of American Food Materials" in an *Office of Experiment Stations Bulletin*. This was the first compendium of his calorimetric analyses and contained the chemical breakdown of no less than 2,600 food items. The compendium charted the fat, carbohydrate, protein and ash content, as well as the caloric value per pound of food for everything from the spinal column of a sturgeon to canned Russian lamprey to vanilla wafers and whortleberries (Atwater, 1896). During the 15-year period between 1895 and 1910, some 350 studies were conducted in federal experiment stations under Atwater's direction. All told, Atwater used the calorimeter to analyze almost 8,000 foodstuffs, publishing the data in various USDA yearbooks and bulletins. Atwater's early dietary studies were the precursor to "official" federal food guides. He was clear that his publications were meant to be a reference for federal dietary standards and he had no reservations about rating the quality of foods based on the proportion of their nutrients:

The information gathered from a study of the composition and nutritive value of foods may be turned to practical account by using it in planning diets for different individuals. . . . By comparing the results of many such investigations it is possible to learn about *how much* of each of the nutrients of common foods is needed by persons of different occupations and habits of life. (Atwater, 1902, p. 32, italics mine)

This statement nicely summarizes the purpose of the next hundred years of nutrition guidance published by the USDA.

Atwater also believed that the scientific analysis of foods had important economic ramifications. In other words, he believed that nutritional ignorance was costly. Hard-working citizens wasted money by selecting decadent and expensive foods that had no more nutritional value than many cheaper ones. With some understanding of food science, caloric composition and good nutrition, Americans could easily spend much less money on the same measured amounts of raw fats, proteins and carbohydrates. Atwater conscientiously defined "cheap food," "healthful food," and "economical food" and stated that the best foods were the ones that yielded the most nutrients for the least money. Distinguishing between good food and bad food then, required an understanding of the scientific composition of various foods, the nutrients they furnish to the human body, and it required calculating a cost/nutrient ratio for each. Economical foods were cheap, healthful, and the most desirable. By conceptualizing the American eater as a rational actor, Atwater justified his message, and its objective criteria for understanding quality. His food guidance assumed that Americans would want to follow his guidelines, would want better nutritional health, and would want to "turn it to practical account." His construction of eaters and his attempts to sway the eating patterns of this fictional population based on scientific reason demonstrate how a discourse of quantification was an ideal language for such a cultural policy.

With such a malleable concept as Atwater's fictional eater, making scientifically or numerically rational arguments seemed commonsensical:

Ten cents spent for beef sirloin at 20 cents a pound buys 0.5 pounds of meat, which contains 0.08 pound of protein, 0.08 pound of fat, and 515 calories of energy, actually available to the body, while the same amount spent for oysters at 35 cents a quart would buy little over half a pound of oysters, containing 0.03 pound of protein, 0.01 pound of fat, 0.02 pound of carbohydrates, and 125 calories of energy; or if spent for cabbage, at 2¼ cents a pound, it would buy

4 pounds, containing 0.05 pound of protein, 0.01 pound of fat, 0.18 pound of carbohydrates, and 460 calories of energy, while of wheat flour at 3 cents a pound it would buy 3½ pounds, containing 0.32 pound if protein, 0.03 pound of fat, 2.45 pounds of carbohydrates, and 5140 calories of energy. Comparing the various materials in this way, it becomes clear that the fresh vegetables are the dearest sources of protein, meats and fish somewhat cheaper, and cereals the cheapest of all; and that oysters and lobsters are the costliest sources of energy, followed by some of the green vegetables and fruits, then the majority of meats, next potatoes, and cheapest of all, the cereals. (Atwater, 1902, p. 42)

Atwater argued that families could minimize poor food choices if they knew how much and what kind of food was essential for the day's diet, and if they knew the most economical foods to select to achieve that diet. A family must first determine their energetic needs for the day. If the woman of the house has "a husband who is engaged in moderately hard muscular work like that of a carpenter or mason or active day laborer," he should take in about 3,500 calories.[20] According to Atwater, "The wife if busy at work with her hands about the house or otherwise, will need perhaps eight-tenths as much," and the four children would together equal three more "men" at moderately hard labor, thus the family requires 1.12 pounds of protein and a fuel value of 14,000 calories (Atwater, 1895, p. 362). The task at hand for Atwater's fictional wife was to select foods that obtained, at the least cost, sufficient proteins, fats, and carbohydrates needed to meet the physical demands of her family. If she could make wise selections and get "abundant nutriments at less cost," she could save a little money for "extra comforts for the family" or for the savings bank.

Applying scientific principles to make an economic argument for the selection of certain foods over others added another numeric dimension to food. The conception of food as energy value was undergoing a transformation into food as a calculated ratio between energy value and financial value. Selecting the right foods now required calculation on two levels. First, the caloric needs of the household had to be determined: food purchases coming into the house had to equal the energetic output of its members. Second, food purchases had to be sound fiscal selections so that the amount of energy and nutrients in the pantry was "economical." The remedy for the evil of overspending was to be found, according to federal publications, "in an understanding of the elementary facts regarding food and nutrition and in the acceptance of the doctrine that economy is not only respectable but honorable" (Atwater, 1902, p. 45).

The enumeration of food allowed its quality to be judged in terms of the ratio of its parsimony and nutritional bounty. Numerically calorifying food allowed for a kind of conflation of quality and quantity—the quality of an eater could be judged easily or compared on the basis of caloric or nutritive content of their diet. Once the method for studying food was established as quantitative, and the knowledge produced easily communicated, reproduced, and compared, a "dietary study" became a routine experiment among USDA scientists. The dietary study examined eating patterns of large populations defined by geography, socioeconomic status, or culture. These studies neutralized social or regional gastronomic acumen, and assisted in the quantitative retooling of food and its relationship to the human body. Atwater pioneered such dietary studies at his experiment station in Connecticut and subsequently encouraged hundreds of these studies at various experiment stations around the country. Because quantification allowed for fast and easy comparisons between and among diets of a variety of communities across the nation, these studies formed the basis for the qualitative judgment of the soundness of one's daily regime. Because the quality of a diet was defined in quantitative terms this rendered the societal patterns of the Yale crew team, the immigrant French Canadian family, and the fruitarian unimportant.[21]

The caloric and nutrient intake circumscribed social conditions and the quality of life of the people in Atwater's studies. The introduction of quantity as an inherent quality to American food and the human act of eating normalized personal gastronomic preferences and allowed eaters, and their food, to be ranked, counted, and measured. According to the USDA, while everyone differed in the amounts and proportions of food they needed to eat, in the actual practice of eating "we are apt to be influenced too much by taste, that is, by the dictates of the palate; we are prone to let natural instinct be overruled by acquired appetite; and we neglect the teachings of experience. We need to observe our diet and its effects more carefully, and *regulate appetite by reason*" (Atwater, 1895, p. 368, emphasis mine). The establishment of these kinds of studies was a fundamental first step in establishing a national and normalized American diet. At the semantic level, a discourse of quantification made gastronomic knowledge impersonal and devoid of any social, cultural, or geographic influences. The implementation and use of reason and rationality shifted a discourse of food and eating from taste and experience to calculation and equation. This shift allowed for the quantitative judgment of eating practices, not the qualitative judgment of those practices, and made possible an "American" dietary tradition (one that would be invented in the 20th century).

But it would take time for this discourse of quantification to solidify itself. Judgments of food and eating practices in America remained deeply cultural throughout the 19th century, despite the advent of nutrition science. Root and de Rochemont (1976) argue that foreign observers of the American diet during this period claimed that American food was "not good" and notable only for its abundance (p. 132). This observation and judgment issued from two important factors: First, the American diet during this period was thought to be monotonous, bland, and heavy because of its reliance on pork, corn, and potatoes. Second, herbs and spices were used sparsely, which meant food had little flavor (McIntosh, 1995, p. 80). Although many aspects of the American diet were seasonal and geographically diverse during this time, the abundance of corn and pork along with a limited range of cooking techniques meant that any American culinary tradition was thought to be poor at best (Jones, 1981). What is notable about this time period, however, is the lack of a robust way of talking about the relationship between diet and health. Qualitative judgments were based on taste (and diet was understood in terms of taste) not nutritional value.

The 19th century was also marked by an enormous influx of immigrants who brought with them their own eating habits (Jones, 1981). But even with these new eating habits, the British cultural heritage carried forward from the eighteenth century helped to solidify an "American" diet during this period (McWilliams, 2005). In both the 18th and 19th centuries, it was the British culinary tradition that most influenced what and how Americans ate, and most directly allowed for qualitative judgments about food (Levenstein, 2003). Because of a certain form of eurocentrism many foods that could grow quite easily in American soil were ignored until they were accepted in Europe (Levenstein, 2003). From this perspective, what was good was European. What made America unique culturally was the abundance of food on the table—otherwise, it was not until the 20th century that America would escape its British heritage. Again, however, what is notable is the lack of a fully articulated connection between diet and health, and instead qualitative judgments were made for cultural and class reasons.

Applying quantification to food and the American eater, a process facilitated by the calorimeter's production of numbers, allowed the USDA to promote gastro-fiscal responsibility, dietary morality, and rational consumer action in the face of these broader cultural trends. The calorimeter was a technology that revealed to USDA scientists the thermogenic functions of the human body, and how the body consumed its comestible fuel. It is this application that represents the launch of the semantic coalescence of quality and quantity of American food. After the development of nutrition, once-moralistic terms like "good" and "bad" become enumerated and objectified in discussions of food. The virtue of numbers and, as Atwater put it, "reason" in the American diet is that they have rigorous certainty, a formulaic method, and the ability to reduce qualitative social patterns to data. The post-calorimeter applications of the quantification of food represent the federal government's complete acceptance of the rules and language of science as the knowledge foundation for an American diet. In the official USDA nutrition guides that become popular publications beginning in the 1910s we see the further development and adoption of a discourse of quantification.

Ted Porter (1995) argues that producing knowledge through objective measurement "was not simply a link to theory, but a technology for managing events and an ethic that structured and gave meaning to scientific practice" (p. 72). The implementation of the methods of quantification validated the USDA as a rigorous political organization guided by objective scientific ideals. Objectivity meant the rule of law, not of men. Because the USDA established and encouraged the ethos of science, and the USDA was the federal body governing American food, this ethos permeated the communication of federal science to the general public. The craft of farming, with its reliance on a practical understanding of the land, was pushed out of favor by the rise of the professional federal scientist. The pattern of academic meritocracy that afforded federal scientists a stamp of superiority over uncredentialed opinion was repeating itself in many arenas of American life at the time, and it did not pass agriculture by. This organizational matrix, that could predict, count, and produce knowledge that was insulated from public debate, disenfranchised the public farmer.

The calorimeter, the data it produced, and the general work at the early experiment stations all certified a new ontological status for food. It is in and through these technologies and numbers that food's essential nature was called into being. Therefore, this early history of nutrition nicely demonstrates how a new reality is manufactured and comes to replace an old reality. Every food item came to signify so much more than it could before the calorimeter, and this refiguring of food made the work in subsequent food guides possible and made the search for more knowledge about the scientific benefits of specific foods necessary. Without the ontological shift made possible by the calorimeter, it is difficult to see how the kinds of knowledge claims made in later food guides would have been possible. In any case, the numbers produced by Atwater signify much more than an abstract quantity. These numbers create a deep set of associations between food and other sets of numbers. In other words, these numbers create a self-referential system wherein numbers begin to refer to other numbers. As such, they trope food by turning our attention away from taste toward this artificially constructed, alternative reality. It is this process of turning, that one witnesses in the charts Atwater produced, that is the major effect of early nutrition research. Once our attention is turned away from the food itself and toward the chemical composition of the food, a whole new world is made far more important, valuable, and real than the world of personal, subjective, or cultural opinions. Over the course of the 20th century the calorie would become the essential signifier of the nature of a food. This new signifier was the major resource in refiguring food and certifying food's "true" nature.

As an authoritative political organization that flaunted its professional status, the USDA attempted to neutralize public opinion about food by the use of a discourse of quantification. This could mean anything from a farmer's knowledge of the right time to harvest his peaches, a homemaker's knowledge of what foods her family enjoyed most, or an immigrant's knowledge of the cultural traditions of eating certain foods on given occasions. These ideas and practices did not have an official space, like the experiment station, or voice, like the *ESR*, and so they became opinions that lacked the scientific rigor the USDA claimed to possess. By normalizing these opinions about food, by establishing official spaces and discourses with which to test and perfect agricultural practices, the USDA tried to establish itself as the *only* source of knowledge about food. The USDA's work with experiment stations is an example of what has become a common collusion between science, congressional politics, and universities. Over the course of the 20th century state-sponsored funding of science in America became a normal practice, and the outcome of such practices, as this case shows, is often an officially, state-sanctioned perspective on a particular scientific/political issue. In other words, it becomes difficult to distinguish the science from the politics (Savage, 1999). In establishing itself as the only source of knowledge about food, the USDA then presented that knowledge to a discursively controlled and normalized public. This public was now quantified and devoid of qualitative cultural differences like taste, habit, experience, or culture. In some ways, this would help "Americanize" the immigrant populations of the 19th century and replace the British culinary tradition that remained dominant throughout that century (McWilliams, 2005).

In addition to the shift in authority from farmer to scientist, a transformation occurred with the advent of calorimetry, when both food and eating developed an abstract, yet implicit, numeric quality. While counting quantities of foods in weights or liquid volumes was nothing new, these quantities did not describe the nature of the food itself. What makes this application of the language of calorimetry to food important is that the quantitative values of a food became its codified and concretized qualities inherent in the food. While a "pound" of apples was brought into existence by a weight scale, the measurement of the "pound" had little to do with the apple itself. However, the measurable nutritional qualities: calories, fats, carbohydrates, and the like became intrinsic qualities of the apple. These quantities, and established constants like the Atwater units, were impervious to social or temporal influence. The truth about food could be spoken using this language of numbers. National nutrition directives emerging from the USDA now had a discourse that was uninfluenced by people, regions, or cultures. Quantification has been called "a social technology—crucial for managing people and nature" (Porter, 1995, p. 50). In the case of enumerated American food, this social technology, born of policy and reared by science, shows how we came to understand food through amounts, numbers, and quantitative comparisons. The taste of the food and our personal likes and dislikes were normalized through this discourse of quantification and as a result, our knowledge of food became nonexperiential and standardized. The quality of our diet became quantities. Our epistemological framework for food became empirical, economic, and numeric. Put simply, understanding the *what* of a food became inextricably bound with understanding the *how much* of the food—this is a drastic ontological shift. It is also a shift that would, over the course of the next 100 years, help to erode the influence of taste, tradition, culture, and experience from decisions about what to eat.

Chapter Two

Reading Federal Nutrition Guides

Quantification as Communication Strategy

In a USDA *Farmers' Bulletin*, Dr. Atwater stated: "the main question is how to use [ordinary food materials] in the kinds and proportions fitted to the actual needs of the body" (1902, p. 38). Public educational material published by the USDA since the 1902 bulletin has focused on answering Atwater's question. Knowing groups of foods by their scientific function and the amount one ought to eat was fundamental to knowing the proper way to eat. Statements like these constructed a scientific alternative to the principle of taste. From the first official food guide in 1917, good food and good food practices came from knowing "how much," and the USDA continuously framed eating as a quantitative and empirical endeavor through the publication of several food guides. These guides often used timely commonplaces that encouraged the reader to think of food as a remedy for social problems. Addressing these social problems, however, meant talking about food in a quantitative manner. The USDA-published food guides provided the forum for the enumeration of food and attempted to popularize and socialize a discourse that had previously been reserved for scientists. By concurrently constructing and solving problems using a discourse of quantification, the USDA created a web of self-referential numbers that reinforced their importance and their discursive dominance.

The USDA's construction and resolution of situations using scientific language made a subjective language of experience or quality absent from federal food policies. Science provided the apparatus for defining a situation, solving problems, and determining standards. In and through the food guides, the USDA attempted to validate and legitimate a discourse of quantification, and it encouraged a quantitative foundation for understanding quality food. For example, the 1917 guide used the rhetoric of need and encouraged households to determine their labor output in order to fuel themselves at work. Food guides published after World War II used a language of moderation and control to legislate proper serving size to address the proliferation of processed fattening foods and an expanding American waistline. Each commonplace pointed to themes familiar to the public during that era. Whether the public was encouraged to eat for frugality during the economic hardship in the Depression, or to eat to keep disease at bay in the post-WWII era, each guide used quantitative arguments that encouraged Americans to follow an empirically determined pattern of eating.

The USDA's default mode of communication about food was a discourse of quantification, and it was this discourse that facilitated the epistemological shift that made quality a quantity. In this chapter, I examine the USDA food guides' messages and outline how these messages encourage the uptake and application of a discourse of quantification. My concern in this chapter is not whether the food guides were successful in teaching the American population about food and nutrition. Rather, this chapter will examine the ways the USDA attempted to address the vast audience of Americans, the language it employed to do so, and the effects it hoped it would have. These federal documents point to the development of a sophisticated language game that certified some claims as true and discounted other claims. One's capacity to perform within such a language game became indicative of one's health.

The food guides acted as a teaching tool for the USDA, but in order for the tools to teach effectively, they needed to employ messages with social resonance. Thus, the messages generated by the guides, in addition to being rooted in a discourse of quantification, were situational, regional, and timely. Themes of authority, knowledge, and objectivity were the frameworks for each guide, but the manner in which these themes emerged, and were used to persuade, changed depending upon the social climate at the time. Each food guide had particular discursive and rhetorical features that attempted to speak to Americans. What was consistent throughout these guides is the refinement of, and reliance on, a discourse of quantification to encourage readers to make judgments about food. By approaching the USDA food guides as teaching tools the assumptions are that social parameters determined what people ought to know about food, but the disciplinary foundations for that knowledge were scientific quantities.

Over the years, the discourse of quantification became increasingly self-referential, and numbers became referents to other numbers, standards, and norms. As scientists at the USDA were able to count vitamins, minerals, and the chemical structure of fats, a secondary discourse of quantification developed. This secondary discourse occurred when quantities (already established as intrinsic qualities of foods) became further qualified through quantitative language of scale or degree. As techniques for measuring the chemical constituents of food became more precise, scientists could determine how much calcium, vitamin D, or niacin a food contained, and they could determine how much of those nutrients were required or necessary for a healthy American. This secondary discourse of quantification gave rise to legislation and regulation of what to eat with standards like the Recommended Daily Allowance (RDA) or the serving size. These sets of numbers allowed people to judge a food's quality based on where its numbers fell in relation to the numeric federal standard. Once an RDA for calcium was established, one could determine whether a food containing calcium was a *good* or *bad* source by whether it contained *enough* or *too little* of the particular element. This secondary discourse of quantification was fundamental to functionalizing foods based on their numeric portfolio. Science determined how much of a particular nutrient was enough, or good for us, and reason became a constitutive part of eating.

The measurable quantities of these micronutrients and the interplay between primary and secondary discourses of quantification gave rise to such concepts as the "average" family's dietary needs and the "standard serving size," both determined and employed by the USDA in their food guides. A secondary discourse of quantification acted in two ways. First, the dietary standards homogenized Americans into large groups delineated only by age and sex. By producing numeric guidelines for how *everyone* should eat, the guides demonstrated that their concern was that America's eating patterns measure up to their standards, and not reflect seasonality, personal tastes, or cultural rituals. The nutritionally sound status quo ate precisely according to the guide. Second, the production of these numbers demonstrated the USDA's commitment to science and quantification as their own, and only, means of communication about food. The ability to produce sets of values using increasingly technological means of experimentation minimized the number of federal authorities on food to those intimately involved with science and nutrition. The processes of normalization and standardization through a secondary discourse of quantification gave the food guides unique units to present their message of nutrition. Determining the quality of a food came to rest upon more than fats, calories, and proteins. The USDA created a glut of numbers that determined a food's "goodness" by quantifying vitamins, trace minerals, and stereoisomers of lipids, and by asserting that certain quantities of these substances were necessary for a sound body.

Ultimately, the food guides presented social amelioration as the justification for heeding nutritional advice. Each guide intimated that the public should eat in a particular way to help alleviate a pressing social issue. Learning to eat according to scientific principles, and understanding food through a series of numbers, would facilitate the eater's achieving whatever social goal the food guide purported to have. This chapter will deal with past food guides, each in turn. Beginning with the first guide in 1917, I will examine the social context that grounded each guide, and the themes that each guide used to encourage particular eating habits.[1]

How to Select Foods:
What the Body Needs—Food Guidance in 1917

In 1917, Caroline Hunt, a specialist in food preparation and use at the Bureau of Home Economics, wrote the first USDA food buying guide entitled *How to Select Foods: What the Body Needs*. This guide obviously emerged directly from Atwater's research: "Evidently what a person who plans meals ought to know is what things the body needs in its food and how these needs can be filled by the ordinary food materials" (Hunt, 1917, p. 3). The stated goal of the guide was to "give a simple method of selecting and combining food materials to provide an adequate, attractive, and economical diet" (preface). Evidently, the diet of the American public was somehow inadequate, unattractive, and financially wasteful. At the turn of the 20th century, cooking and cleaning had become the lexical domain of a discourse of quantification. Domesticity "expanded into an objective body of knowledge that had to be actively pursued" (Shapiro, 2001, p. 7). This objective body of knowledge formed the basis for the study of home economics. The founder of the home economics movement was Ellen Swallow Richards, whom Caroline Hunt revered, who ran a community experiment station in Boston that was "fully grounded on the latest principles of science," and whose goal it was to "educate the people in the best habits of food preparation and nutrition" (p. 6).

Messages of standardization, order, and efficiency were consistently present in the scientific approach to domestic space. In addition, scientific advice also became a hallmark of contemporary motherhood, or "scientific motherhood" as Rima Apple (2006) calls it, in the early 20th century. Instead of relying on instinct and common sense to raise children, mothers were expected to acquire the specialized knowledge of experts in order to raise their families healthfully, normally, and appropriately. In other words, to be a good mother required none of the natural, inborn abilities to care for children that were often thought to be commonplace aspects of maternal love, and instead required women to allow scientific and medical experts to intervene in family life to guide parenting practices. The 20th century's obsessive and anxious concern with proper parenting techniques seems to nicely parallel the concomitant anxiety over food and eating practices. In both cases, parents and eaters seem to have accepted the notion that only expert scientific advice could provide the best guide to making decisions for the family. Such a transition is a move away from other forms of knowledge, experience, and authority in the name of scientific progress. Early 20th century journals such as *Infant Care, Babyhood*, and *American Motherhood* all sought to deliver scientific advice, including advice on proper eating habits. These efforts to communicate the results of scientific experimentation to mothers were centered in the same land grant universities that subsidized nutrition research, and in some cases conducted by the same home economists.

Paralleling the changes to motherhood, therefore, the Bureau of Home Economics had been working closely with USDA scientists, who sought an efficient and simple way to teach the public about food. Teaching people the *proper* way to eat was of great concern to community experiment stations and USDA extension co-ops (who employed home economists) because it offered immediate access to the homes of the nation. The home economics movement considered the dinner table a rapid way in for reforming Americans' eating patterns. Everyone had to eat, and the USDA's goal was to tell them how, what, and how much. This first food guide in 1917 established the pragmatic value of food that was simple, clean, and wholesome. Food ought to meet the family's "fuel value" per day, and the food guide encouraged consumption in proper quantities, ratios, and combinations. The guide shows a photo of a bounty of eggs, milk, bread, fish, beef, and a basket of fruits and vegetables, and it outlines a sample meal for a sample family (a man, woman, and three children):

Food materials such as those shown in the pictures may be combined into three meals in many ways. The following meals are given not because they are recommended above many others that might be used but simply to show that such foods can be combined into dishes that are commonly used in American homes. The meals here suggested would supply the following substances in about the right proportions to keep the family in healthful condition and to make the food taste good, providing they were well prepared. (Hunt, 1917, pp. 5–6)[2]

Here proportion comes before taste and efficiency is the prize to be won by following the guide.

How to Select Foods uses "need" as the theme around which to structure the problem of filling human physiological requirements and the maintenance of human labor output. The guide "tells very simply what the body needs to obtain from its food for building its tissues, keeping it in good working order, and providing it with fuel or energy for its muscular work. It shows in a general way how the different food materials meet these needs and groups them according to their uses in the body" (preface). The German model of the "body as machine" that was imported by Atwater at the turn of the century remained as a permanent fixture in this USDA guide. The guide contrasted these "needs" for tissue building, strength, and muscular work with the irrational appetite and the unreliability of hunger and personal tastes. It warns that in determining what one ought to eat "appetite is not always a safe guide," and "neither can hunger and its satisfaction always be relied on" (3). One of Hunt's main concerns in the guide is that the nutritive demands of the hard laborer be met, and the home economist took great pains to categorize what each type of laborer, woman, and child needed:

> The exact amount which each person needs depends upon age, sex, size, and amount of work done with the muscles. An elderly person, or one of quiet habits, needs less food than a vigorous young one; a large person more than a small one; a man more than a woman; grown persons more than children; and a farmer working in the hayfield, a mechanic, or a football player more than a man who sits at his desk all day. (11)

By learning how to select foods according to the calculable physical output of this individual, and by cooking like they do in common "American homes" the empirical needs of the family would be better met than if they followed an individual's appetite, hunger, or satisfaction.

For those families who did not follow the principles of the guide, Hunt was not optimistic:

> It is believed that it is impossible to plan the meals for a family wisely without at least as much knowledge of how different kinds of food serve the body as this bulletin has given and that the safest short cut to good planning lies in considering foods in the five groups here described. (12)

Wisdom, as Hunt defines it, comes from a body of knowledge—knowing the functions of food, quantities that define food's functions, and human caloric requirements. Meeting the empirical needs of the family becomes the goal for the home cook, not feeding their yens, or creating eminently tasty dishes. The cultural subjects defined by "age, sex, size and amount of work done with muscles" ought not to be satisfied with the meal because it tasted good, but rather because proper food selection met their needs.

The establishment of the five food groups—fruits and vegetables, meat and meat substitutes, starches, sugars and fats—in the 1917 guide show the influence of Wilbur Atwater, who happened to be the father of Helen Atwater, Caroline Hunt's coauthor. The 1917 guide used Atwater's numeric nutrition research and shaped it for public consumption. Using Atwater's fat, protein, and carbohydrate caloric allotments and calorimetry research, Hunt grouped foods based on chemical composition and their scientific function in the body. The groups, Hunt claimed, "will be helpful for the housekeeper to form the habit of thinking of the many different kinds of food which she handles. . . . If the housekeeper will consult [the groups] in planning meals until she has learned where each kind of food belongs, she will have taken the first step toward providing a diet which will supply all the food needs of her family" (pp. 8–9). Here, Hunt outlines the importance of method in meal planning—thus, the food guide begins to foster a particular understanding of quality food. Following the method of food grouping for meal planning reassured the housekeeper that her meals would be simple, correct, and nourishing. The guide encouraged the "wise" housekeeper to "think of foods according to their group" during meal planning, shopping, and curing and canning for the winter (pp. 10–11).

The notion of "fuel value" used in the guide also served as a first attempt to conceptualize food solely in terms of numbers (p. 4). One needed to calculate how much of particular groups of food one needed in order to have enough energy for the day. The guide lays out several "sample meals" for families (p. 6). One such meal specifies that a family of five should eat 2 pounds of fruit (which, according to the guide, is the equivalent of 4 medium-sized oranges, or 5 medium-sized apples, or 6–8 ounces of dried fruit, or 20–25 prunes), 2 pints of cooked cereal, 5 cups of milk, 8 slices of bread, 1½ ounces of butter, and 2 eggs. The justification for these, relatively crude quantitative suggestions, was articulated in terms of what foods "should provide" for the proper functioning of the body (p. 6). The relative ratio of fruit to meat in one's diet, for example, was an essential calculation to make because it let one know if all of one's body's needs had been met. This perspective on food, as fuel for the body, was a first step in refiguring food because it demanded that calculations be made to determine the best diet. It would take more research for the discourse of quantification, here displayed in primitive form, to develop in sophistication, but the basic formula and basic demand for more quantitative knowledge were both in place in this first guide.

In order to make people aware of their nutritional deficiencies, and to point to edible solutions to the deficiencies in their diets, *How to Select Foods* roots the process of food selection in nutritional science. It simplified the eating process by placing foods into five groups. According to Hunt, if all of the food groups are "represented regularly in the meals," then the family's nutritional needs are sure to be met. The food groups charted in the 1917 guide made food's pragmatic value explicit. Grouping a food imparted it with reason. In the light of such a move, one could know how to eat a food in a particular way, at what particular time to eat a food, and what kinds of people really needed that food. The method of food selection, therefore, was based on the presence of a number of groups on the dinner plate. Each group served a quantifiable physical need of a stratum of American society and demonstrated the first food guide's commitment to eating by numbers. *How to Select Foods* recasts the dinner plate, food shopping and food preparation into a science experiment, foisting upon the housekeeper a new language and a new knowledge about food.

The tenor and theme of this guide also dovetailed with the continuing concerns over the future food supply and whether or not the world would be able to feed an ever-expanding population (Belasco, 2006). The worry, beginning in the 1790s with Thomas Malthus's population studies, was that population growth would outrun food supply. With waves of immigrants and overcrowded cities, the 1920s witnessed a return to the Malthusian concern with a potential crisis of overpopulation. Chemistry would be the solution to this pending crisis. Sir William Crookes, writing in 1917 (the year of Hunt's guide), went so far as to claim that "starvation will be averted through the laboratory" (qtd. in Davis, 1932, p. 754). Encouraged by the success of technological inventions from electricity and automobiles to plastic, margarine, and artificial nitrates, synthetic foods were thought to be the best hope for the growing population. If these synthetic foods were to feed the nation, however, they must be able to deliver the right amount of calories and nutrients. Studies and predictions of population statistics were often accompanied by calculations of the total number of calories that would be needed for a population (in the 1930s, William Hale contended that mankind required 6 trillion calories a day). These calculations obviously belong to a discourse of quantification, and the potential problem of overpopulation could only be solved through scientific advances that made more quantities of food available. But calories were not the only concern—cost and other nutritional characteristics would also become essential to the construction of dietary advice offered by the federal government.

Diets at Four Levels of Nutritive Content and Cost— The 1933 Food Guide

Between the first food guide in 1917 and *Diets at Four Levels of Nutritive Content and Cost,* published in 1933, there were sweeping changes in both the social and agricultural landscape of America (Mcelvaine, 1993). When Hazel Stiebeling, the senior food economist at the USDA, set to writing this guide in 1933 for the USDA circular, the "average American home" faced widespread unemployment, breadlines, and hunger marches. For example, 25,000 people participated in a hunger march through Chicago on October 31, 1932, to protest cuts in relief payments (Cohen, 1991). President Herbert Hoover's refusal to enact compulsory crop reduction left silos full of grain to rot on American farms, and Hoover's disdain for federal assistance, and a decline in the export markets, left farmers dealing with surpluses that depressed food prices (Saloutos, 1982; Kirkendall, 1975). The ideology of order, process, and progress that reigned during Caroline Hunt's food guide in 1917 had been replaced with a profound sense of insecurity and uncertainty about the future. In the face of the breadlines and malnutrition, the USDA stood ever more firmly behind the scientific principles of nutrition. The response to the dire economic situation was to use a discourse of quantification as a solution to the economic uncertainty. The 1933 guide begins: "The present economic situation has focused attention upon national as well as individual planning for the best use of food resources. Basic to any such planning is knowledge of food values, of the nutritional needs of the body, and of the relation of food to health" (Stiebeling, 1933, p. 1). While the social and economic situation in 1933 was radically different from that of 1917, the discourse employed by the 1933 food guide remained the same. Just as the 1917 food guide could help you determine your needs and then fill them, the Depression-era guide helped you determine your economic status in order to plan your meals around it. It was easy for the 1933 food guide to apply the additional quantitative dimension of determining monetary value for nutrients because the 1917 guide had already grouped and functionalized food.

From 1929 to 1933 the average family income had dropped by 40%, and in 1932 more than a quarter of all American households did not have a single employed worker. By 1933, 30% of the U.S. labor force was unemployed (Nixon and Samuelson, 1940). During the 1920s, however, the idea that poor peoples' inadequate diets were the result of their ignorance of nutritional science and not their low income had become a commonplace assumption (Levenstein, 1993, p. 6). The 1933 guide, therefore, made scientific arguments to encourage food selection and meal planning using food groups and ratios of nutrients to cost. Nutrient value for dollar became an important factor for the grocer who wanted to know which nutritionally worthy foods appeared in the USDA diets of all economic echelons of society. Additionally, those buying food wanted a good economic and nutritional return on the foods they could afford:

> Both the *consumer* and the *producer* are demanding information on food selection based on this new knowledge of food values and nutritional needs. The consumer, interested in getting good returns for what he can afford to spend, wishes to have this information interpreted at several economic levels. The producer on his part, wants to know how much of different foods may well appear in the diets of different consumer groups, and to what extent consumption may rise or fall as the economic situation changes. (p. 1)

These demands, articulated in the introduction of the food guide, led the USDA to develop four levels of diets that were based on the economic status of the reader. Each level provided plans for weekly and yearly quantities of foods that furnished the nutritive requirements of families. Numbers and science remained at the fore—charts, graphs and food groups (there were now 12) encouraged the reader to approach food as a quantitative solution to an economic problem. Economics determined which diet plan a family should follow: the restricted diet for emergency use, the adequate diet at *minimum* cost, the adequate diet at *moderate* cost, or the liberal diet in which cash outlay was not a factor in food selection. Whether someone ate the restricted diet or the liberal diet was unimportant, the science of nutrition guaranteed that the nutritive content of each diet met with the minimum daily requirements of the body. These numeric portfolios allowed for the food guide to rate the quality of a food based on the nutritional return for economic expenditure.

Stiebeling's guide is far more quantitatively sophisticated and elaborate than Hunt's guide. Over the course of 60 pages, and countless graphs and charts, the central goal of the guide is to articulate the quantities of specified nutrients one needed based of the four different kinds of diets. Because of the variability in food costs, Stiebeling makes a whole set of quantitative recommendations so that one could acquire all the calories one needed. For example, in any given year those on a restricted diet should eat 240 pounds of flour and 8 dozen eggs while those on a liberal diet should eat only 100 pounds of flour and 30 dozen eggs (p. 2). These differences were also calculated in terms of percentages, which meant that 43% of a restricted diet should be flour and 5% lean meat, fish, and eggs, while 15% of a liberal diet should be flour and 21% lean meat, fish, and eggs (p. 3). These quantities are justified by reference to the average price per pound of particular foods (which added an additional quantitative layer of information to the guide). After price per pound was determined, each food was then analyzed for the amount of calories, protein, calcium, phosphorus, iron, and vitamins A, B, and C per pound. This allowed Stiebeling to analyze the economic and fuel value differences between, for example, fresh tomatoes and canned tomatoes and make recommendations in the light of that data. Finally, the guide determined the "proportion of calories derived from specified types of food" and the "approximate retail money value" of specific foods as well as the "proportion" of one's retail money that should be used for specific foods (p. 15). These calculations were the constitutive features of the guide's dietary recommendations. Clearly for the USDA, the discourse of quantification that Hunt first began using in 1917 had emerged as the default mode of understanding food and making judgments about what one ought to eat, and that discourse was now elaborate and complicated.

Stiebeling also included charts indicating "nutrients purchasable for one cent." Using these charts, she allotted different foods to different diets. Grain products, dried beans, and potatoes are especially important in low-cost diets. Other vegetables, fruits, lean meat, fish, and eggs are more prominent in liberal diets (p. 10). While someone eating according to the liberal diet could finance 165 pounds of lean meat, poultry, or fish and consume only 100 pounds of flours and cereals a year, someone on the restricted or adequate diet for minimum cost scaled their meat consumption down to around 40 pounds and increased their starch consumption to 240 pounds per year. As the guide points out:

> [B]readstuffs and cereals yield for the expenditure excellent returns on calories, protein, phosphorus, and iron. Most fats are important primarily as low- or moderate-cost sources of energy in concentrated form. They help to make a high-cereal diet palatable and give a "staying quality" to the food eaten. (p. 10)

The 1933 guide constructs a solid relationship between food and economics, but food, as the guide conceives of it, is a set of nutritive quantities

and not considered a locus for human interaction, taste, or cultural celebration. Though Stiebeling is concerned with a food's palatability, the
food's goodness is derived from its nutritional return. The USDA's use of
a discourse of quantification, and the food guide's encouragement to learn
food values, both economic and nutritive, establishes two things in this
case. First, a scientific understanding of food can save money. The wise
consumer knows how many nutrients each food contains and (once they
have determined at which level they ought to eat) can prevent wasteful
spending on nutrients in luxurious foods, when those same nutrients exist
in cheaper comestibles. Second, the 1933 guide further institutionalizes
the notion that the quality of the food is measured in quantitative terms.
"Good" food was judged by numbers, dollars, and nutrients and not by
personal judgment or taste.[3]

The 1933 Chicago Fair reinforced these claims and demonstrated the
connections between this form of federal dietary advice and the changes
happening to the agricultural industry. The motto of the fair was "Science
Finds—Industry Applies—Man Conforms." The belief was that the march
of machinery together with advances in chemistry would drive the family
farmer out of business in favor of the full-scale application of chemistry
to all phases of the food chain. Scientific food production was made possible by advances in the discourse of quantification. With more elaborate
descriptions of the mysterious inner chemical constitution of foods, the
belief that man could alter and improve the work of nature seemed to
gain ever-stronger traction. Thus the industrial changes to the food chain
underway at this time and the continued pursuit of synthetic, functional
foods were a product of the success of the discourse of quantification that
the 1933 guide enshrined and promoted.

Vitamins and the Advent of a
Secondary Discourse of Quantification

Atwater, Richards, Stiebeling, and others had focused most closely on the
economics of food, arguing that efficient spending on food could maintain
good health. The home economics movement used these ideas to appeal
to middle-class women concerned about health, housework, and frugality.
But the years between the 1917 guide and the 1933 guide extended the
discourse of quantification and the scientific approach to food beyond
these concerns. Scientific data about food's chemical composition, and the
quantities of nutrients associated with food, increased markedly between
the 1917 guide and the 1933 guide. This increase in the volume of available food data occurred for two reasons. First, the apparatus for testing

foods became more sensitive and the determination of trace elements like iron, phosphorous, and calcium became more accessible to more people. Second, and more importantly, the discovery of the importance of vitamins and the establishment of a relationship between the intake of certain foods and the incidence of disease led to new advances in nutrition research. The mounting evidence that linked low vitamin intake and the increased incidence of deficiency diseases caused a shift in the way food was perceived to work in the body. This shift further developed the discourse of quantification by making measurements of already scientized food quantities the basis for judgment of food. This double layer of measurement functionalized food as more than just fuel. The quantities of nutrients, minerals, and vitamins in food assumed an active role in preventing disease and causing good health.[4]

Wilbur Atwater's model of the body, upon which the 1917 food guide interpreted nutrition, focused on the notion of a closed thermodynamic system that produced energy based on the practical economy of food. In Atwater's model of nutrition, what went into the body worked to sustain the muscles and provide energy for physical output. Vitamin research began in America in 1913, with Wisconsin biochemist Elmer McCollum reporting a fat-soluble growth-promoting substance in egg yolk and butter. This substance, which they called "fat-soluble A"—later vitamin A—differed from the water-soluble "vitamine" that Polish biochemist Casimir Funk had found to prevent beriberi, vitamin B.

The discovery of vitamins and their biological application represent a pivotal moment in the functionalization of food. The Atwater model showed food to function as energy and muscular sustenance. The discovery of vitamins showed that not all proteins, carbohydrates, or fats were equal in their nutritional content. Some foods were empirically "better" than others. While Atwater parsed out the differences between fats, carbohydrates, and proteins, and argued that the body needed ratios of all three dietary components to build muscle and provide energy, McCollum's work in vitamins asserted that not all kinds of foods in the Atwater groups were created equal. Certain proteins provided more or less of the disease-preventing vitamins than others, and certain carbohydrates could provide both energy and muscle-building proteins.

McCollum rejected the simplicity of Atwater's model because it "did not make it possible to have a qualitative, as distinct from a merely quantitative, evaluation of foodstuffs and, therefore, of diets" (Cravens, 1996, p. 143). A chemist like Atwater was only concerned with the quantity of foods taken into the body; McCollum's biologically informed research could investigate the quality of what was inside a food. But McCollum's understanding of quality food depended on the number of vitamins and nutrients it contained and supplied to the body. McCollum's notion of quality was as quantitative as the model he rejected. What mattered in a food was the biological function of its constitutive microscopic nutrients, not the chemical makeup of the food itself.

The measurable vitamin content of food allowed the USDA to establish required quantities of specific foods in emergency, adequate, and liberal diets, as well as establish the quality of food by constructing a ratio of furnished nutrients and cost. Functionalizing food by grading its quality in terms of its quantity of vitamins established a secondary discourse of quantification. As vitamin content became an important quantity in foods, food became an instrument of nourishment by Atwater's units and an instrument of disease prevention by its constituent vitamins. Not only did the USDA want American eaters to concern themselves with taking in sufficient calories, they had to make sure that the calories they ate were from "quality" sources—that is, rich in quantities of vitamins. These quantities allowed the USDA to establish dietary intake standards, quantities of food that were necessary to keep Americans healthy and disease-free. These standards, reflected in the diets, were the precursor to the formally established and published Recommended Daily Allowances that appeared in the next decade. These RDAs fortified the role of a discourse of quantification because they worked to normalize food habits and eating patterns with a set of edible numbers toward which all Americans were to strive.

By 1933, a scientific knowledge of food was considered basic to proper eating, and *Diets at Four Levels of Nutritive Content and Cost* uses a discourse of quantification, functionalized foods, and minimum requirements of vitamins and minerals to fortify the Depression-driven themes of planning and need. Because the family's diet plan was economic, this guide uses nutritive value for dollar as the criterion for quality food. Scientized and quantified food was thus the means with which to address the Depression's economic situation. This food guide also begins to add a self-referential quantitative discourse. The eater compared foods' numbers to generate judgments about quality based on those numeric comparisons. This enumeration of already quantified foods marks the beginning of a secondary discourse of quantification. The more numeric knowledge the USDA produced the more authority they granted science to become the epistemological foundation of good food. The extra stratum of quantities in the discovery of vitamins made it important that those purchasing and preparing the meal analyze it carefully before eating. The quality of a food depended on its caloric composition, how much it cost, and how many nutrients it contained.

These advances in the discourse of quantification also made the pursuit and dream of functional foods more likely. For example, Dow

Chemical's William Hale's books, *Chemistry Triumphant* (1932) and *The Farm Chemurgic: Farmward the Start of Destiny Lights Our Way* (1934), imagined the radical reorganization of the farm through the synthetic improvement of grains, meat, and produce. Eventually, so engineers and scientists like Hale thought, the constitutive features of food like proteins could just be synthesized directly instead of from eating steaks. This kind of direct chemical production of nutrients for human consumption was the dream of agricultural science during this period, and it was a dream made possible by a discourse of quantification and its ability to refigure food within the imaginary of the American public. Federal dietary guidance made these dreams seem normal and not outlandish or crazy. Obviously, the future of food was just a matter of synthetic chemicals that we could ingest without the hassle of eating so that we received the nutrients we needed. The food industry was pursuing the simplification of the equation and federal dietary advice would provide the recommendations for what chemical ought to be synthetically produced and consumed.

The 1940s Recommended Allowances and the Wartime Basic Seven

In January 1941, President Franklin D. Roosevelt called the National Nutrition Conference for Defense to generate some information about the nutritional status of the nation. America was at war and the United States needed strong healthy troops to aid the allies. Reports, however, described American health as grim at best. The Depression had taken a huge physical toll on Americans and, unless America was better nourished, the war effort would be hampered greatly. The surgeon general, Thomas Parran, warned that "forty percent of the American population are not properly fed. The ill-health results mean a slowing down of industrial production, a danger to military strength, and a lowering of the morale of millions."[5]

In wartime, good food was considered to be fundamental to national defense, and the beginning of the draft heightened the worry that malnourished men could not win the war. President Roosevelt asked the Committee on Food and Nutrition, a 41-member branch of the National Research Council, to quantify exactly how much of each known nutrient Americans needed to be in good health. Once science determined how much people ought to be eating to be healthy, the U.S. government could establish standards to which people could compare their diets. If Americans were to be strong as a nation, these standards were critical when they planned their meals and ate their food. The chair of this committee, Dr.

Russell Wilder of the Mayo Clinic, appointed a subcommittee of three home economists—Lydia Roberts of the University of Chicago, Helen Mitchell, a veteran of Kellogg's sanitarium in Battle Creek, Michigan, and Hazel Stiebeling of the Bureau of Home Economics—to determine exactly how much and how many nutrients Americans needed. Over the next several months, the committee evaluated, scrutinized, and arrived at the "Recommended Daily Allowances for Specific Nutrients," a table that specified quantities of nutrients whose intake prevented nutritional deficiencies and nutrition-related disease.[6] Arriving at this set of numbers was not an easy task. Experiments in nutrition literature had widely varying numbers, and several nutrition experts had differing opinions as to what the daily recommendation ought to be. The foreword in the *Proceedings of the National Nutrition Conference for Defense* hinted in diplomatic political speech that the RDAs were a compromise to many committee members.

> The values here as given thus represent the combined judgment of nutrition authorities in various parts of the country. This does not mean, of course, that every contributor would fully agree with all of the figures as given. It does mean, however, that the values are ones they were willing to accept tentatively, until standards derived from more exact data can be obtained. The term "Recommended Allowances" rather than "Standards" was adopted by the Committee to avoid any implication of finality.[7]

Such a move ensured the continued production of these guides, along with the continued federal funding of nutrition research.

The numbers generated by the committee did not report minimums, the least amount of each nutrient you needed to be in good health. Instead, the chart's "daily allowances" reported numbers that exceeded the minimum standard by about 30%. The conflicting opinions of nutritional scientists provided the committee with such a wide range of data that in order to prevent dissension, the numbers of the RDAs were both high enough to assuage scientists with generous standards and low enough to prevent discord among those with lower estimates (Levenstein, 1993, pp. 65–66). The chart mapped out arrays of RDAs for men, women, and children. At a glance, one could determine their requisite daily number of calories, protein, and grams of calcium based on their age and activity level. After consulting the chart, a lactating woman could feel happy knowing that if she consumed 23 milligrams of nicotinic acid that she had met her recommended daily allowance. The establishment of the RDAs, released in May of 1941 at the National Nutrition Conference for Defense, was a critical moment in the development of nutrition research and American food guidance.

The RDAs represented another means for the USDA to introduce a discourse of quantification into the practice of eating, and another way for the American eater to be quantified. The RDAs forced the aggregate eater to compare herself with sets of numbers and judge her own quality based upon whether she falls above or below those standards. The quantitative self-policing encouraged the eater to think of themselves in terms of age, sex, correct caloric intake, or levels of thiamin. By publishing the RDAs, the USDA attempted to redefine the eater's inadequacies in terms of numbers and have the eater manage those deficiencies by eating for quantitative reasons. This helped form a kind of ethically incomplete cultural subject (Miller, 1993).

While the generation of these numbers by the committee satisfied President Roosevelt and validated the data of (some) nutritional scientists, it marked an important moment in the development of a discourse of quantification. After the establishment of an "official" dietary standard for various nutrients in the American diet, there was a definitive line in the sand of sustenance. A food's quality could be ranked based on quantities of nutrients, and a quantitative discourse could be generated by comparing the numbers of nutrients in a food and the standard number required for a healthy American—now one deemed food good or bad depending on whether or not it could provide specified amounts of nutrients to the American attempting to meet her daily allowance. The RDAs helped to further the epistemological shift that quantified quality, and they helped the proliferation of a secondary discourse of quantification by encouraging comparison between people and the chart. Americans needed to eat more or less of particular nutrients in order to become good or better, that is, closer to the quantified RDA. The Recommended Daily Allowance created a fictionalized numeric ideal of a healthy public: millions of people who, if they followed government suggestions, could be healthy Americans. The publication distributed by the USDA dubbed the RDAs "a yardstick for good nutrition."[8]

In addition to homogenizing and categorizing the American eater, the RDAs further delegitimated taste as an important factor in food. Prior food guides encouraged Americans to count foods to counteract disease, to fill a need, or to save money. Apart from determining daily energy requirements, often determined by what job the eater held, the enumeration of the eating process lies solely in the food itself. Each food had an important numeric portfolio, and that portfolio determined what and when we should eat—not what we felt like eating or what tasted good to us. Past USDA guides had enumerated food but had never before quantified the human body's relationship to food—or crafted so strong a relationship between the selection of quality food and the makeup of a healthy or quality individual. The RDAs constructed a nutritional problem in numeric terms: in order to measure up, one must eat to this numeric goal to be a healthy American. The RDAs stripped subjectivity from American eaters, and made eaters manage themselves and their meals through calculation instead of craving. As such, it was not surprising that the federal benchmark did not measure satiety, satisfaction, pleasure, taste, or the enjoyment of food. Gone too are the economic and employment-based judgment about how much to eat. The RDAs represent the moment in which the person, in the process of eating, falls away, and the judgment of the goodness of a meal and the goodness of an American becomes a measurement.

In 1943 the USDA published the *National Wartime Food Guide* to accompany the Recommended Daily Allowances. The guide stated that its nutritional structure would provide the lion's share of the RDAs but that the individual would have to supplement servings from the basic seven food groups in order to meet the day's caloric needs. The guide was spartan in its content and simple in its message. In the throes of the war effort the *National Wartime Food Guide* told Americans that "The U.S. Needs Us Strong—Eat the Basic Seven Every Day." Using the discourse of quantification, the *Wartime Food Guide* used the theme of strength to encourage numeric eating. A meal that provided strength had foods from all of the basic seven food groups. Reducing the number of food groups from twelve in 1933 to seven in 1943 allowed the food groups to correspond loosely to the recommended nutrients in the newly established RDAs. The wartime guide gave green and yellow vegetables, decent sources of iron and riboflavin, their own group separate from oranges, tomatoes, and cabbage, which provided vitamin C and the "potatoes and other vegetables and fruits" group whose highlight, the spud, was a source of nicotinic acid. Groups four, five, and six were dairy, proteins, and complex carbohydrates that provided calcium, vitamin D, and thiamine. "Butter and fortified margarine" had its own group, owing to the fact that it had "added Vitamin A." The food guide did not dictate exactly how many of each group one should eat in a day, only that "to keep healthy and strong, use *some* food from each of the seven groups every day."

In 1946 the USDA published an updated version of the wartime guide that eliminated the explicit references to strength. However, the guide was otherwise exactly the same with a nuclear family walking hand-in-hand happily into the future. Both of these versions of the "Basic 7 Food Groups" were considerably shorter than the previous guides and provided less written instruction. Instead of several pages of explanatory text included in previous guides, this guide gave lists of foods in each

THE BASIC 7 FOOD GROUPS

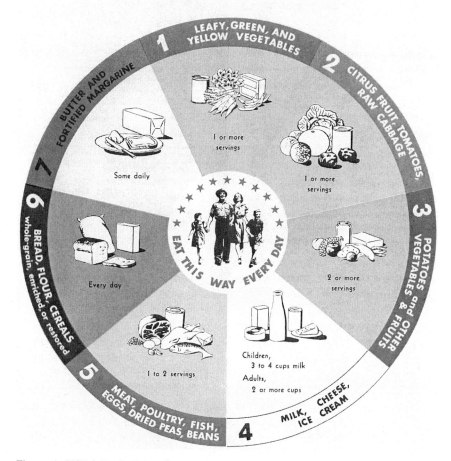

Figure 1. USDA Basic 7 Food Groups, 1946. National Food Guide USDA Leaflet 288, 1946. (Source: USDA)

food group, and summarized its message with a picture of a pie-like representation of the seven groups, where each food group was pictured radiating out from a smiling family at the center of the pie. The wartime guide was the first to shift formats from lengthy and explanatory text to iconographic images that had pictures represent what to eat. While previous food guides had addressed food preparation, and included recipes or daily meals, this guide made no mention of how to prepare any of the food listed or how to plan the daily meals to adhere to the guidance. In a sense, the *National Wartime Food Guide* and the 1946 *Basic 7 Food Groups* delivered information about food in a way that was completely objective while completely ignoring the practices of eating. Proper food and eating do not need pages of explanatory text; they need simple equations with lists of variables and a pictographic reminder to stick to the "Basic 7." These structural changes mark the discursive pattern for the food guides to come. Symbols come to replace syntax as the guides became less discursive and more diagrammatical.

The development of the Recommended Daily Allowance and the pared down *National Wartime Food Guide* and the more generic 1946 *Basic 7 Food Groups* guide represent the governmental response to the exigency of World War II. The message was clear and simple: food could fortify Americans and heeding the government's recommendations about nutrient intake could guarantee that you would be a strong and contributing member of American society and the war effort. Using the war as an authorizing theme to encourage certain practices in the American household was common. In addition to these guides' connection to the American war efforts, many food companies (or companies involved with food preparation or storage) attempted to link their messages to the war. Everything from Florida grapefruit "Rich in Victory Vitamin C" to Wilson meat that "protects your table," to Crosley household appliances whose spokeswoman claimed that "planning meals is the way I can fight" used the war in their advertising campaigns. Books with titles like *Nutrition, The Armor of Robust Health* (which explained the benefits of bread and enrichment) and *Food, A Weapon for Victory* appeared on the shelves. In 1941 the U.S. government formed the War Food Administration that was responsible for maintaining good American nutritional health during wartime. The WFA published a series of pamphlets on food rationing, food preservation and canning, and planting victory gardens. Because war was on the minds of the American government, and their publications, it is no surprise that the USDA's food guide used war as the reason for both learning about the scientific functions of food and adhering to the numeric standards of eating.

Using the RDAs as a numeric foundation, the *Wartime Food Guide* and the generic 1946 *Basic 7 Food Groups* give a simple scheme for achieving strength, the exigent theme of the war. Eating by groups, pictures and numbers no longer needed explanation or justification. The Basic 7 chart was an epistemological tool that made clear that the only kind of knowledge about food was empirical, and that reliance on the empirical could help you make decisions about "what to grow in your garden, what to store and can, and what other foods to raise besides vegetables." If you were out at a restaurant "remember the seven food groups when choosing food," and use the basic seven "in planning meals to be served in lunchrooms or to be carried in the lunch box by school children, war workers and others."[9] Wherever and whatever you were doing with food, the guide encouraged you to think of the groups, the explanatory diagram, and the cause. Good food practices were calculated, and quantified food could fortify America at war.

The discourse of quantification and the scientific ethos extended into other aspects of wartime food concerns as well. During the war waves of panic buying of certain foods encouraged the government to develop a food-rationing program. In May 1942, the government issued ration books with the most sought after items: coffee, sugar, and meat. Rumors of shortages of these ingredients created actual shortages due to hoarding and thus forced the government into the rationing program. While Americans responded negatively toward the democratic ethic of rationing, they responded in an overwhelmingly positive way to the government's request to grow their own food. Planting a victory garden to ensure success in Europe was a way for the government to use bellicose topoi and encourage a measured approach to food (Bentley, 1998). By late 1943, 40% of American vegetables were grown in the home, canned, and preserved. Because the government claimed that food was the first line of defense in the war effort, it was not only what you ate that kept you strong and healthy, but also how food was obtained and controlled that was important as well. The U.S. government printing office published, in 1943, a 16-volume compendium, "The U.S. Government campaign to promote the production, sharing and proper use of food," which outlined the "overall food problem" and covered the victory gardens 1943 campaign, the meat-rationing time schedule, as well as the campaign against black markets in meat. For their authority, the practices relied on the objectivity of a discourse of quantification. Rationing is itself a technique of quantification, and such techniques were natural extensions of the kind of work being done in the official dietary advice offered by the federal government. To "eat for victory," to use Amy Bentley's (1998) phrase, required a working commitment to a discourse of quantification as a common sense approach to food and eating just as nutrition and health did.

The end of World War II also brought ominous population predictions about the number of future Americans and the possibility of starvation and malnutrition. But politics and industry continued its commitment to the scientific ethos and its belief that science would be able to meet the demands of a growing population. By 1949 all Corn Belt acreage was planted using hybrid corn seeds that produced higher yields. This was a clear example of both the faith in science to meet the pressing demands of a future population *and* the importance of quantification in judging

quality—more corn is, of course, better. But the threats of future population booms also coincided with a newfound awareness of the rest of the
world's problems with starvation and hunger. New statistics demonstrated
percentage of calories from grain, meat, and milk for different countries
and found a correlation between wealth and consumption of meat. Many
worried that with more people America might become a grain-eating
nation and not a meat-eating nation—this, of course, meant that future
Americans would not enjoy the standard of living that they did at that
time (Belasco, 2006, pp. 46–47). In this context, every new agricultural
technology was thought of as a way to increase the global supply of
foods (particularly animal foods). Abundance meant luxury, and thus the
machinery of American industry and government was put in the service
of producing more, not better, food.

The Essentials of an Adequate Diet—The 1956 Food Guide

In 1956, Louise Page and Esther Phipard of the Household Economics
Research Branch of the USDA wrote *Essentials of the Adequate Diet*, the
food guide that replaced the Basic Seven. Post–World War II America was
booming and the servicemen from "the best-fed army in history" returned
from the war wider, heavier, and accustomed to colossal army portions of
food.[10] During the war America was asked to give up their food for the
GIs overseas, "after the men in the armed forces have been taken care
of, the rest of us will all go on getting three square meals a day." Thus,
in wartime, the average American consumed about 125 pounds of meat
per year and the American soldier consumed about 360 pounds, most of
which was beef (Dyson, 2000). The best-fed army became accustomed
to a super-sized diet based on the basic seven food groups, and returned
home expecting the same sort of salubrious meals. After food guides that
counseled America during times of need, planning, and sacrifice, the 1956
guide could loosen its quantitative restrictions on how much America
needed to eat: the suggestion was as much as it wanted.[11]

By 1956 the field of food processing was rapidly expanding and
synthetic chemical food additives and preservatives made their way
into American supermarkets, extending shelf lives, improving mouth
feel, and making food more colorful than ever. Science and technology
were making more food and more types of food available to Americans
than ever before. Many of these new foods, and new eye-appealing packaging, arrived on the supermarket shelves thanks to wartime experiments
in factory preparations and food dehydration. Fast food and prepared,
frozen meals like the TV dinner became parts of the edible fare avail-

able to Americans. Kraft Foods introduced the luminous orange Cheez Whiz in 1953, Carnation Company introduced instant nonfat dry milk in 1954 and the first McDonald's opened in 1955. By 1956, the days of rationing food, and rationing money to pay for food, were gone, and the USDA's attitude was that Americans had a bounty of affordable food at their disposal.

The USDA's 1956 guide responded to this theoretical smorgasbord by attempting to simplify food guidance, and by giving the consumers as much flexibility in "good" food choice as they could without compromising federal nutrition standards. The USDA thought that the wartime guide that divided food into seven groups was too complex for peacetime. The design of the 1956 guide came from the urge to simplify the quantified process of eating by reducing the number of food groups in a nutritious diet. The USDA moved around fruits and vegetables and lumped all of them into one group, butter lost its group status and the Basic Seven became the Basic Four. As such, food guidance became less directive and more suggestive. The Basic Four touted the new guide meant as a *"foundation* for a good diet . . . whether or not other dietary needs are met depends on choices made within food groups and also on the kinds of foods selected to provide the remaining calories." Foods that were considered luxury items in the past were expected to play a significant role in supplementing the foundation:

> To round out the meals and to satisfy the appetite many people will use more of these foods (in each group) and everyone will use foods not specified—butter, margarine, other fats, oils, sugars and unenriched refined grain products. Thus these foods are a part of daily meals, even though they are not stressed in the food plan. (Page and Phipard, 1956, p. 1)

The guide begins by announcing how many cups of milk one needed, and how many servings each of meat, breads or cereals, and vegetables or fruit. These quantities are then elaborated in terms of what percentage of one's daily intake of calories, protein, calcium, iron, vitamin A, thiamine, riboflavin, niacin, and vitamin C a particular food group contributed. For example, a child should have 3 to 4 cups of milk, which contributed about 25% of one's daily intake of protein. The guide then develops an elaborate point system so that one could calculate how many points of milk one had consumed in a day. Extensive charts list the point values of many different foods so that one could make sure one was getting enough calories, protein, and so forth. The end of the guide recommends quantities for daily meal plans so as to insure that one knew exactly how much of each group should be consumed in relation to the other groups in a balanced meal. These quantities were all one really needed to know about particular foods in order to eat well (at least according to the USDA).

Essentials of an Adequate Diet stressed that America had enough food in the country to furnish every individual with their recommended nutrients, but that people ought to eat what is adequate, that is, neither too much nor too little, if they were to maintain good health. Americans could be adequate if they ate the *minimum* number of servings from the newly established food groups. Unlike previous guides, the 1956 guide did not recommend replacements or substitutions the eater needed to make, nor did it mention economic aspects of food selection. The guide urged people to recognize the importance of following the food guide's groups when constructing their meal, and to acknowledge the proper serving of each food group, but it also highlighted the flexibility of the new plan:

> Each of the *broad* food groups listed in the daily food plan has a special job to do in helping toward an adequate diet. In the number of servings specified and with the choices indicated, these food groups together furnish all or a major share of the calcium, protein, iron, vitamins A and C and the B-vitamins recommended by nutritionists. (p. 1)

The USDA's use of a theme of adequacy in the food guide, and their prescription of a serving size to define "adequate," illustrated a new concern. Past food guides concerned themselves with helping people make wise, scientifically validated food choices when their choices, for a number of reasons, were limited. By 1956, the USDA assumed that the availability of all types of foods was widespread, and the concern was that overindulgence, not under-indulgence, in the supermarket's bounty could be a problem. That all Americans had access to sufficient food, and would hence engage in overeating, was not the case. Despite rapid agricultural mechanization of food processing and harvesting, as well as advances in food distribution, many Americans, most of who lived in the rural South and Appalachia, suffered from severe malnutrition, which cut along socioeconomic and racial lines. This problem was largely ignored by the U.S. government until Robert Kennedy (D-New York) visited Jackson, Mississippi, and saw that thousands of African American farm workers and sharecroppers had been displaced from their farmland by mechanization and were near starvation or surviving on one meal a day. This visit occurred in 1967, 11 years after the USDA introduced the Basic Four food guide, and it was only after Kennedy's visit that food and hunger became a political issue in Lyndon Johnson's War on Poverty.

The USDA's determination of what "adequate" meant relied on the scientific data that the home economists used in the 1940s to generate the Recommended Daily Allowances. Their quest for simplification, however, meant that having the public learn the RDAs was not feasible. What resulted in the 1956 guide was an entirely new quantitative lexicon for food. In lieu of having people learn about milligrams or International Units (IU) of particular vitamins, minerals, or essential nutrients, the guide allotted each food a number of points, where one point represented a certain quantity of a nutrient. The development of a point system (which the USDA jettisoned after the 1956 guide) and the suggestion of a serving size added more abstract numeric dimensions to the diet. While the eater could choose from a greater number of options, and from fewer defined groups, they had to allot points to each food and divide foods into serving sizes. Although foods may occupy the same group, some were better than others, and this depended on their point portfolio:

> This point system provides a way to check daily food choices to make sure that the food group as a whole furnishes the amount of a key nutrient expected of it. It has the added advantages of dealing with simple whole numbers, and of employing the same term—"point"—for each nutrient. . . . Although foods within each group are much alike in food value, they vary in amounts of nutrients provided by a serving. To help in making choices, foods in each group have been rated in points to show how they compare as sources of a key nutrient. For each nutrient, 20 points represents the minimum counted on from a particular food group and corresponds to nearly half or more of the day's allowance for an average adult. (Page and Phipard, 1956, p. 2)

The point system encouraged people to check that their food choices supplied the nutrients they expected, and that they were not just eating random quantities from each food group.

Concurrent with the development of the point system, the USDA established a standard for what they deemed a single serving of each food ought to look like. Like the points, the standard serving size was informed by the quantity of RDAs that a particular food group supplied. For example, the USDA judged a serving of the meat group, important for "the amounts and quality of the protein" it provided, as 1 ounce, which provided around 7 grams of protein, or 5 points. The guide recommended 2 or more daily servings from the meat group and since the daily goal for protein intake was around 60 grams, the eater had to heed the "or more" condition in order to be nutritionally acceptable.

The most obvious and simple way of appraising the meal record is to count the servings of various types of food and to compare the number with the minimum suggested in some food plan or guide. The most reliable method of judging dietary adequacy is to calculate from food value tables the nutrients provided by the diet and to compare the results with recommended allowances. (p. 16)

The point system gave eaters a very simple way to keep score of their meal and to use a numeric measurement as the arbiter for the goodness of their food. Because this method of counting was, according to the USDA, the "most reliable," and the "most obvious and simple way of appraising the meal," there was no need to seek alternatives to the point system, or the discourse that formed its foundation.

In postwar America numbers and science continued to govern eating patterns. The *Essentials of an Adequate Diet* was, according to its mission statement, a "foundation diet." Following the guide, the serving sizes and the number of points or servings per day would provide the eater with the "essentials," which the USDA expected the eater to supplement with additional foods to "round out meals and satisfy the appetite" (p. 1). If one ate according to the Basic Four, they would be in numeric nutritional compliance, and they would receive the major share of calories, protein, and nutrients to furnish their energy and health needs. However, to round out the diet, the USDA expected that many people would use more of the recommended number of servings a day, as well as use foods not specified by the guide: "butter, margarine, other fats, oils, sugars, and unenriched refined grain products." These "other" foods were not quantified for nutrients or serving size, nor was there a discourse of quantification that addressed what might be enough, too much, or too little of these foods.

The 1956 guide followed the same discursive patterns as the other guides and used a quantitative discourse to judge the quality of food. But the guide does acknowledge that certain foods have unquantifiable features—many of which make food *taste* good. *Essentials of an Adequate Diet* quantified those foods that had specific functions in the body and that furnished certain dietary needs. It was around the Basic Four food groups of breads, meat, milk, and fruits and vegetables that a secondary discourse of quantification existed and that serving sizes were prescribed. The "other" foods: fats, oils, sugars, and unenriched refined grain products, which "helped make meals flavorful and satisfying" and added only calories to the diet, were (in 1956) unquantified, portionless, and hailed as contributors to the pleasure of the meal (pp. 12–13). To be an average, adequate, and healthy American, you would eat certain foods from certain food groups, count your points per day, and score your meals according to this point tally. But to satisfy yourself, the USDA expected that you supplement your "adequate" meal with pleasurable foods, and this pleasure was unbridled, uncounted, and immeasurable:

> These "other" foods are frequently combined with the suggested foods in mixed dishes, baked goods, desserts, and other recipe dishes. Fats, oils, and sugars are also added to many foods during preparation and at the table to enhance flavor and improve appetite appeal. (p. 1)

Because quality was defined in quantitative terms and through the scientific process, the USDA could easily define good food. But the USDA could not count what Americans ate for pleasure or flavor. In the 1950s, food with little nutritional or scientific value was immune to a discourse of quantification.

Fifty Years of Federal Food Guidance

The continued use of quantification and the reliance on scientific findings to guide nutrition policy during these 50 years was a clear example of the larger trend of deference to expertise in American politics. The ability of a profession, and nutrition science had now clearly become a profession, to identify and solve complex problems was often the justification for this deference. It is during these same 50 years that the social sciences as a profession emerged (Haskell, 2000). In the light of immigration, urbanization, and industrialization, a professional class of scientists developed a set of tools to solve social problems that arose from these factors, particularly in medicine (Starr, 1982). What the disparate social sciences shared was their approach to problem solving—an approach grounded on specialized, and often quantitative, language and knowledge. Through specialization and knowledge production, these professional scientists were able to acquire considerable authority for themselves. The story of the USDA food guides is an example of that trend.

This trend also included the advent of professional organizations and a political transition away from party politics and toward the emergence of an "administrative state" (Schudson, 1999; Galambos, 1982). Experts relying on a discourse of quantification were essential to the management of this administrative state, from economists guiding rate-setting commissions to doctors managing public health initiatives and agricultural scientists promoting efficient farming techniques. The Progressive Era, from which much nutrition science and advice emerged, marked the beginning of the broader integration of scientific knowledge into the federal government and policy-making institutions, and this trend was solidified throughout these 50 years. Hunter Dupree goes so far as to label the Department of Agriculture during the Progressive Era a "predominant" agency of science (Dupree, 1963). The Great Depression and World War II played a significant role in expanding this alignment into all areas of science and politics and pushed experts and the state closer together (Balogh, 1991). Physics, for example, would become central to America's war effort, and the development of nuclear science demonstrated the relevance of scientific knowledge and the importance of the link between expertise and political governance.

Franklin Delano Roosevelt's presidency was an excellent demonstration of the intersection between quantification, science, expertise, and politics (Kirkendall, 1966). Relying on academics interested in economic and industrial planning (A. A. Berle, Raymond Moley, and Rexford Tugwell to name three), F. D. R. established substantive and important links between government and academic professionals. Formalized institutions like the Temporary Economic Committee and the National Resources Planning Board allowed social scientists to use quantitative evidence for social problems. The time period between the Progressive Era and World War II saw the advent and solidification of a symbiotic relationship between professional experts, well versed in discourses of quantification, and the public institutions of governance (Price, 1965). The war, so many thought, illustrated in clear fashion that expertise could produce results in the face of crises (Rourke, 1969). Thus, the period between 1945 and 1970 was marked by a drive to produce more expert, quantitative knowledge, which resulted in the expansion of the research university (Newman, 1981).

Perhaps the best indication of the broader influence of discourses of quantification was the creation of the "New Class." In the 1960s, Daniel Bell noted that society was moving from blue collar to white collar, with new institutions that were "intellectual," with important political implications. Political decisions would increasingly become dependent on experts of this new class, which would limit the ability of ideology to influence politics. The attitude in the Kennedy White House, according to Arthur Schlesinger Jr., was "that public policy is no longer a matter of ideology but of technocratic management" (Dickinson, 1984, pp. 265–266). The 50 years of nutrition advice produced by the USDA is one small strand in the larger story of the inexorable expansion of the role of expertise, quantification, and scientific knowledge in guiding public life in America. Across the board, the consistent assumption was that specialization and professionalization could provide the kind of data critical for rendering good judgments about complex issues. The only thing that may seem odd in this story is that choosing what to eat was considered a complex issue worthy of such extensive scientific attention.

Through 50 years of federal food guidance, crafted with a discourse of quantification, that set out to make judgments about the quality of a food based on numeric measurements, no guide ventured to address the pleasurable aspects of eating, the taste of certain foods, or what it meant to have a "good" meal in the qualitative sense of the word. Because the USDA's work never concerned tasting food, flavor, or the eating experience, it lacked a language to describe that experience. Foods that tasted good fell out of the bounds of quantitative limitation because the USDA could not tell you how much pleasure you could have. When the USDA had to address a new subset of foods that had little scientifically proven nutritional value, they were unable to do it because they were bound by an empirical discourse that could not describe the subjective experience of eating.

From a rhetoric of need in the 1917 food guide, to a rhetoric of adequacy in 1956, each USDA food guide used layers of quantitative discourse to address particular domestic social situations. Learning about how, what, and why to eat in a scientific or numeric fashion became the goal of the food guides. Enumerated food selection represented economic frugality during the Depression, the Recommended Daily Allowances encouraged the public to eat to meet certain federal recommendations, thus fortifying the public during times of war; serving sizes and points were the pragmatic functionalization of food so that the host of nutrients could be more easily counted at each meal according to the portion size. In each case, scientific knowledge was used to different social ends. However, the means to that end was the same: communication about food through a discourse of quantification. The food guides' messages encouraged people to learn about and use knowledge of science to make the best decisions about what to eat.

These food guides give us a method for understanding the meaning of *quality*: a meaning defined in quantitative terms. Each new food guide introduced new themes to contextualize and deliver new information about food. Adhering to the letter and spirit of enumerated food by counting food groups, vitamins, nutrients, or pennies committed the household to solving a pressing problem of the era. This method required scientific knowledge, elaborate calculations and structured meals that rested on a quantitative lexicon and terms like "adequacy," "balance," and "sufficiency." If the reader aspired to be a "common American home" (1917), to "keep the U.S. strong" (1943), or to live "within the framework of food habits and food supplies of the United States" (1956), then that reader relied on the USDA's epistemic machinery to inculcate a discourse of quantification. Enumerated food, and the folks who counted it, could contribute to American society in meaningful ways. In each case, however, the underlying message did not depart from the established manner of quantitative communication.

The USDA's use of timely themes suggests particular courses of action to particular groups of numerically defined individuals. Food guides, federal dietary allowances, and numerated concepts like serving sizes and points created types of eaters, all of whom had to use numbers to define themselves and their meals. The USDA relied on the food guides to have Americans manage their own eating practices. The discourse of quantification facilitated this management because it had a normalizing effect on the population. Where you live, your cultural or family history, or your personal likes and dislikes were unimportant to the USDA. A discourse of quantification could not articulate the quality of the experience of eating. And so, these subjective notions and ways of understanding food are repressed by the federal quantified standards and mandates.

Accordingly, the discourse developed in these federal guides served to eradicate the importance of taste in eating and narrow or reduce our conception of health. The implicit, and often explicit, assumptions in the USDA food guides were that an enumerated diet was somehow better than a diet that relied on the whims of human hunger, the ambiguity of the appetite, and the imprecision of the palate. Personal tastes were dismissed as unimportant as increasing data about food gave rise to the creation of food groups, governmental recommendations for nutrient intake, and standard serving sizes. What followed from ignoring the importance of the taste of food was the triumph of objective measurement over subjective judgment.

Chapter Three

The Food Pyramid

Visualizing Quantification

In the latter half of the 1970s a substantial body of scientific research emerged that correlated overconsumption of certain foods to various diseases. Thus, in 1977, the U.S. federal government began to scrutinize the guidance of the Basic Four food groups. It seemed as though Americans were heeding the advice of the old food guide and eating the "minimum number of servings" of the food groups per day. However, while their diets may have been replete with vitamins and minerals, many Americans were going above and beyond the call of nutritional duty and supplementing the foundation diet with considerably more calories than they needed. With American avoirdupois on the rise, the government appointed a Senate Select Committee on Nutrition and Human Needs in 1977 to assess the problems with food guidance and seek solutions. This committee published *Dietary Goals for the United States*, which marked the beginning of the end of dietary advice to eat more.

Although the committee published the *Dietary Goals* in 1977, it was not until 1992 that the suggestions made in the report manifested themselves in a new USDA guide: the Food Guide Pyramid. The Pyramid differed markedly from earlier guides in its message and its appearance. For most of the 20th century, the USDA's main concern was to ensure that the American diet was adequate or sufficient. In order to achieve a numerically defined adequate diet, one had to learn about food groups, serving sizes, and the balance between food intake and energy output. An adequate diet was achieved by consuming the correct proportions and quantities of certain types of food for certain types of people. To ensure that one was getting sufficient amounts of vitamins and vital nutrients the guides recommended consuming *more* than the numeric standards. Servings, food groups, and daily allowances were numbers that constituted minimums; eating these amounts was good, but eating more was better. The dietary goals in the 1977 report reflected a new problem at the American dinner table—more had become too much. Scientists and nutritionists pointed to overconsumption as the cause of a host of diet-related health problems: cardiovascular disease, cancer, and obesity to name three. In response, the USDA and the Department of Health and Human Services began crafting a new nutritional message for the public: eat less. While the new message about food changed from "eat more" to "eat less," the language of the message remained the same: quantitative, numerically self-referential, and validated by science.

New food guides were also faced with having to tell the public that while certain foods may *taste* good, they were not necessarily good for their health. Foods that imparted pleasure to the meal, and were used for "extra calories" in the 1956 guide, were now coming under quantitative scrutiny—for example, butter was bad, sweets and sugars were sinful. Up to this point, the notion of "good" food had been defined by the quantities of scientifically determined nutrients it contained. Judging the quality of food was by measurement, not taste, smell, or pleasure. Because the USDA could not address pleasure, taste, or satisfaction using this discourse, and because the prevailing sense was that America needed to eat more, foods that were nutritionally impoverished but often tasted good were not subject to limitations or standards. The new food guide needed to address these unquantified foods, because they were, scientists believed, a major part of the new problem of American corpulence:

> The simple fact is that our diets have changed radically within the last 50 years, with great and often very harmful effects on our health. Too much fat, too much sugar or salt, can be and are linked directly to heart disease, cancer, obesity, and stroke, among other killer diseases. In all, six of the ten leading causes of death in the United States have been linked to our diet. (*Dietary Goals*, 1977, p. xiii)

In response to the rise in the incidence of American obesity, the new food guide provided gastrostatistics and groups of foods that the eater ought to avoid.

In the 1956 guide "pleasurable additions to meals" were unquantified, either in the number of groups one should consume per day, or in their numeric nutritional portfolio. In the 1992 food guide these previously unquantified foods, mostly fats and sugars, had new numeric standards that the eater needed to fall *below* to be eating right. Foods that were not good for you, or had quantities of undesirable components, were deemed bad. The problem of overconsumption prompted the USDA to quantify "bad," to use a secondary discourse of quantification to encourage the consumption of less bad and more good, and to sharpen the numeric distinctions between more and less. This new guide reconstituted what a good American diet ought to look like and the USDA continued to use science and quantitative language as the epistemological basis for quality food.

In 1992, after 15 years of work, the USDA released the Food Guide Pyramid to the American public. This guide was based on new research and was to serve as the latest nutritional guidance that would replace the outdated Basic Four. The Food Guide Pyramid had revamped food groups and daily servings and serving sizes. For example, "good" foods like fruits, vegetables, and whole grains had sets of numeric goals that America aspired to attain. In addition, the USDA confronted a new question in regard to their strategies for communication: were all of these numbers and food facts too much for Americans to remember? In the early phases of "communication research" to determine the best format for the guide, participants in focus groups complained that they felt bombarded by ever-changing information about which food was good and which was bad.[1] This new guide had a new message, and in order to bring it to consumers the USDA needed a memorable way to convey the new message concerning variety, proportionality, and moderation. The solution was a picture, an illustration of a pyramid that could portray quantitative information and concepts like proportionality. By the time the USDA had arrived at a message for the new guide, it took an additional four years of market research, evaluation of perceived usefulness, and several graphics before they released the pyramid to the public. According to the USDA, "the most important characteristic" of the food pyramid was its shape and the ability of that shape to "communicate the proportionality and moderation concepts" (*USDA's Food Guide*, 1993, p. 28). Instead of rethinking the discourse itself, the USDA codified this language and its myriad concepts into an icon.

This chapter will provide a historical outline of the development of the Food Guide Pyramid and it will outline the developments in government policy leading up to the food pyramid. The USDA demonstrated a deep faith in science in both federal hearings and their selection of consultants and nutrition experts, as well as in the language of the guide. Because the 1992 Food Guide Pyramid addressed a new exigency, the public health of America, the construction of the message required careful attention.

This new nutritional message and the language the USDA employed to articulate this message attracted the attention of a variety of agriculture lobbyists and interest groups. In previous cases, these political players had no problem with the language of the guides. Past federal policy was concerned with diseases of deficiency, problems that America could solve by eating more of everything. Thus, the food industries offered no resistance to simplified messages like "eating more is good." Eating more meant, for the food producers, that they could sell more. When the 1977 Senate Select Committee reviewed the American diet and attributed a variety of disease of excess to certain foods like sweets, fats, and red meat, those respective industries became more vocal about how the USDA enumerated foods. Because corporate and policy interests diverged, some industries, the American beef industry in particular, became very interested in the language the USDA used.

Changing the Message from Too Little to Too Much

Ironically, the impetus behind the creation of the Senate Select Committee on Nutrition and Human Needs in 1968, the governmental body that released the *Dietary Goals for the United States* in 1977 that reported that Americans needed to "reduce their consumption" of fats, calories, and sugars, was a *CBS Reports* episode entitled "Hunger in America."[2] In fact, in the documents of the legislative history of the Senate Select Committee, the entire transcript of the show is adjacent to the page that contains the Senate Resolution 281, the resolution that created the committee.[3] Formed in response to the crisis of hunger in America, the committee was to:

> Establish a coordinated program or programs which will assure every United States resident adequate food, medical assistance and other basic necessities of life and health and shall contain appropriate procedures for congressional consideration and oversight of such coordinated programs.[4]

Despite growing research about the perils of excess food already afoot in American dietary circles, the fear persisted in the U.S. government that many Americans were not getting enough nutritious foods and that they needed *more* food to supply all of the nutrients required for good health. At the first session of the committee in December of 1968, the CBS documentary and the Citizens Board of Inquiry report "Hunger U.S.A." were mentioned in the welcoming statement by Senator George McGovern.

McGovern called these reports "revelations" and looked to the "best minds in the country—experts" to help "end hunger in America."[5] The first expert the committee called to speak was Dr. Jean Mayer, a professor of nutrition at Harvard University: "I would like to point out first that if there is any science that can be termed an 'American science' it has been nutrition . . . there is no country on earth which has contributed as much to our general knowledge of nutrition as has the United States" (*Hearings*, 1969, p. 11). In his address, Mayer mentions Wilbur Atwater, the country's agricultural extension programs, and the pioneering programs of the USDA in cereal enrichment before he gets to the substance of his speech. The malnutrition of the poor is a problem, but "a great deal of our present health problems are due to nutrition even among the rich; with the present emphasis of American medicine on curative rather than on preventative medicine, I am sorry to say that little is done about this aspect" (*Hearings*, 1969, p. 12).

Mayer points to the rise of cardiovascular disease as the reason that a country with such colossal spending on health care had seen little increase in life expectancy. A prescient Mayer criticizes high saturated fat intake, a slothful and gluttonous public, and "presidential fitness committees which have been farces so far" as target problems for this committee to solve. In the questions that followed, a skeptical Senator Charles Goodell asked, "You consider *nutrition* is a prime factor in this, producing this situation in this country?" Mayer replied, "I think the two prime factors are the type of diet we eat and the lack of physical exercise. I think we are the most physically inactive country, particularly our men, on the face of the earth" (p. 34).

By 1977 when the committee issued its first nutrition mission for America, hunger had fallen off the senatorial radar as the pressing issue for the select committee. The committee's report, *Dietary Goals for the United States*, known among nutritional scientists as the McGovern report, stated that American eating patterns were a critical public health concern, and that the recommendations of the *Dietary Goals* were based on scientific evidence that would "provide guidance for making personal decisions about one's diet." Despite being formed in response to the rhetoric of "not enough," the Senate committee was dealing with a health crisis of "too much." Overweight Americans vastly outnumbered hungry ones (p. 34).

The take-home message of the McGovern report was its seven dietary goals for the United States based on "current scientific evidence" (*Dietary Goals*, 1977, p. i). The guidance was not a legislative issue. As McGovern stated in the foreword, it was "rather, [to] provide nutrition knowledge with which Americans can begin to take responsibility for maintaining their health and reducing their risk of illness" (p. iv).[6]

Testimony in the report made by Julius Richmond, MD, the assistant secretary of health, stated:

> Many experts now believe that we have entered a new era in nutrition, when the lack of essential nutrients no longer is the major nutritional problem facing most American people. We believe it is essential to convey to the public the current state of knowledge about the potential benefits of modifying dietary habits. (p. xxxiii)

Scientists and doctors were also called to speculate on the economic savings (in healthcare costs) with a nutritionally improved America. Dr. George Briggs, Berkeley professor of nutrition, estimated a potential annual savings "based on the more conservative end of the range of scientific opinion" at 40 billion dollars (p. 2). The scientific "experts" were encouraging this rhetorical shift from more to less, and the USDA relied on this panel of experts to provide statistics, measurements, and predictions to define the new rhetorical situation.

Of the seven dietary goals in the report, four of them began with the word "reduce," one began with "avoid," and one with the words "limit the intake." The lone goal that began with "increase" was advising the public to increase their consumption of complex carbohydrates and "naturally occurring sugars" (p. 4). A new nutritional paradigm was on the horizon and it was defined by the enumerated discourse now common to food. The *Dietary Goals*' preface reads:

> We believe it is essential to convey to the public the current state of knowledge about the potential benefits of modifying dietary habits, without overstating the benefits that could possibly result from the adoption of alternative dietary practices, such as reducing excessive caloric intake and eating less fat, less sugar, and less salt. (p. xxxiii)

Dietary Goals is widely recognized as the turning point in government food policy.

In *Food Politics*, Marion Nestle (2002) points to the period between 1969 and 1990 as the "shift to 'eat less' " and writes about the political tumult that ensued when the command to eat less became the new message from the USDA. Food historian Harvey Levenstein (1993) called the post–senate Select Committee era the era of "Negative Nutrition" and claimed that the *Dietary Goals* were responsible for a "complete about-face in government nutrition policy" (p. 207). Advice to eat more pleased everyone—the food industry, scientists, the federal government and nutritionists—advice to eat less did not; but when the USDA had to craft a message to counsel America to eat less, there was enormous furor from the American Medical Association and the meat, milk, egg, and sugar industries.

It was not the exigency of the ever-expanding waistline, the widespread inactivity among Americans, or even the rise in rates of coronary heart disease, diabetes, and other chronic ailments that upset the AMA and various food industries. Their distress lay in the wording of the new dietary goals. For example, during the Senate hearings before the release of the *Dietary Goals*, the message to reduce was not appetizing to the meat industry. In one hearing discussing cardiovascular disease, Senator McGovern asked an advisory doctor, Dr. Stamler, how he felt about a lexical change in the message from "decrease consumption of meat" to "increase consumption of lean meat":

> McGOVERN: Dr. Stamler, would you have any objection to modifying the chart to say increase consumption of poultry, fish and veal and other lean meat?
>
> DR. STAMLER: I think it would be excellent.
>
> McGOVERN: I think we ought to do it. One of the problems we are going to bump up against and we already have is that the livestock producers are going to start raising cain about this committee telling people to eat less beef.[7]

In the past, industries rejoiced in the messages of the food guides. Encouraging Americans to eat "enough," "sufficient," and "more" meant that they had to *buy* enough, sufficient, and more. In earlier food guides each food group had a specific purpose ensuring its consumption, food guides listed *minimum* serving numbers per day, and the goal was to use additional "other" foods like fats, sugars, and refined grain products to "bring up the calorie level up to or beyond 100 percent" (Page and Phipard, p. 1). In all earlier food guidance, the rhetorical situation was defined by lack—a lack of nutrients or a lack of calories—and the USDA used a discourse of quantification to both define and solve the problems of paucity by encouraging measured intake of more food. In 1977, the McGovern report pointed to the dangers of this now dated message—more food seemed to indicate more girth, more heart disease, and more cancer. Americans who used to be deficient because they did not eat enough were now deficient because they were eating too much. Federal policy then, in order to address this problem, had to recast the notion of a deficient subject from one of lack to one of excess.

According to past food guides, a "good" food contained quantifiable nutrients, met certain levels of recommended dietary allowances, and provided a known quantity of caloric energy. The 1977 *Dietary Goals* forced an epistemological shift in what constituted quality food. Quantities that had been rhetorically silent for most of the 20th century, now became important determinants of quality and according to the new guidelines, a quantitative "less" became a qualitative "more." A food's content of cholesterol, fats, sodium, and sugars, quantities that had never been considered evidence for judging a food, now needed to be "reduced," "limited," and "decreased." The dietary goals read:

> Reduce the consumption of refined and processed sugars by about 45 percent to account for about 10 percent of total energy intake . . .
> Reduce cholesterol consumption to about 300 mg a day . . .
> Limit the intake of sodium by reducing the intake of salt to about 5 grams a day. (p. 4)[8]

As with the other guides, the new message had numeric yardsticks, but the goal was to fall *below* certain standards and not above. As loathsome as the message may have been to industry, the government and the American eater, using a discourse of quantification to establish new guidelines for what marked a good food was an epistemologically economical thing to do.

The dietary goals of the McGovern report simply made the USDA rethink their list of quality foods. One example states: "With respect to overall fat consumption, it may be useful to follow a strategy of selecting greater numbers of foods that derive 30 percent or less of their calories from fat" (*Dietary Goals*, 1977, p. 4). Accompanying this goal was a table that listed "The Percentage of Calories from Fat in Foods." Desirable foods that would meet the new guideline of "less than 30%" were skinless white chicken meat, water-packed tuna, bread, skim milk cheese, and most breakfast cereals. The fewer calories, fat, or cholesterol a food had, the better the USDA deemed it to be.

This reversal of the desired quantitative quality that constituted good food demonstrated the definition of a new exigency using an already established discourse. The USDA's linguistic framework of quantitative language, which constructed both the problems and solutions of the American diet, remained the default mechanism for communication. By continuing to use science and a discourse of quantification to communicate and organize what to eat and why, the USDA ensured epistemological efficacy. While the message about what to eat had changed, the food guides presented the evidence to eaters in terms they already knew: numbers, quantitative comparisons, and measured objectives. With the USDA's new message about "good" food, eaters had only to renumerate their conceptualization of quality from more to less. The commonplace of quantity made possible the discursive shift from more to less. Because this commonplace relied on the situation to give it content, shifting the definition of quality using quantitative language was easy. By 1977, the new nutritional problem of overconsumption had emerged and the content of the argument of the USDA had changed.

The passage from the *Dietary Goals* forms the explanation for why it is possible that the USDA food guides would use the familiar topic of quantification in its attempts to persuade the public. Science generated trustworthy arguments. Quantification was the commonplace, the discourse that persuaded and buttressed arguments of "authority, usefulness, complexity and bounty," which in turn deepened the "willingness to trust the overall goals of that research" (LaFolette, 1990, pp. 174–175). This was not an unusual practice at the level of American public policy. Robert McNamara, for example, had just been framing his arguments about U.S. military intervention in Vietnam around demands for quantifiable data (Lebow, 2006). At the level of public health, a discourse of quantification was failing the USDA, but at the level of language, that discourse was a success. Changing the message would have been a risky endeavor for the USDA because it would have required introducing another discourse that did not have the same kind of cultural weight as quantification, numbers, and science.

The problem of overconsumption, the shift from more to less in dietary advice, and the new focus on the percentage of fat in particular foods were all part of the context of what has become known as the obesity epidemic in the United States. Over the course of the 1980s and 1990s obesity science became its own branch of nutrition science, replete with a discourse of quantification and a "disease" that relied on that discourse for its existence. The food guide pyramid emerged within the context of this growing concern with obesity. But what the obesity epidemic demonstrates most clearly is that numerical analysis holds the possibility of inventing the diseases that healthy eating would ultimately solve. In other words, obesity is not like other diseases (with clear causes like viruses, tumors, bacteria, or genetic mutations), and so obesity science was left with the task of demonstrating the negative consequences of overeating.

Obesity science, however, did not originate in the 1980s. As part of American nutrition research, the energy-in and energy-out equation that drove the early food guides also provided the grounds for the first studies of obesity. For example, E. E. Cornwall, in 1916, nicely previews some of the central concerns that emerged later in the century:

> It would be an easy matter to calculate the formula for reducing the fuel value of the food intake, if oxidation in the body were always regular and uniform. In such case the amount of reduction would have a caloric value, equal to that of the quantity of body fat which it is desired to burn up. For example, if the reduction in weight desired is at the rate of two pounds a week, which means the combustion daily of about four and a half ounces of body fat, the fuel value of the daily ration would have to be reduced about 1000 calories below the normal for size, age and activity. (p. 601)

Obviously Cornwall is drawing on Atwater's work to speculate on basic weight-loss strategies. However, he also noted, relying on some of Atwater's findings with the room calorimeter, that "variation in oxidation" was common in different subjects with different body types. These variations complicated the energy-in and energy-out equation. In any case, balancing the energy equation was the key to preventing obesity. Beginning with A. W. Pennington's work in the 1950s, as well as general advances in nutrition science regarding fats, vitamins, and minerals, this energy-in and energy-out equation was challenged as a legitimate explanation for obesity (see Gard and Wright, 2005, pp. 80–81). Nutrition science throughout the second half of the 20th century is marked by a seemingly endless series of attempts to explain the causes of obesity, to demonstrate that obesity is a cause of other illnesses, and to recommend strategies for preventing obesity, all in ways that extend beyond the simplicity of the energy-in and energy-out equation. These explanations, demonstrations, and recommendations, however, are all made possible by the discourse of quantification used so simply in Cornwall's work. Moreover, these explanations, demonstrations, and recommendations often come couched in stories of sloth and gluttony, and are not free from ideology or politics. But the use of numbers and statistics has made the morality of obesity seem objective.

The story of the rise of the obesity epidemic, therefore, is equally a story of the triumph of an ideology and politics of quantification. It is a story of ontological and epistemological invention made possible by the common sense view of the value of quantitative assessments. One can begin to see the political and ideological common sense behind the invention of the obesity epidemic in the light of the numbers that are used to define a person as overweight or obese. The surgeon general and the CDC calculates Body Mass Index (BMI) as the primary basis for claiming that obesity is a major health epidemic. The concept of BMI was not, however, originally developed as a tool for judging body fat. In the 1830s, Belgian astronomer Adolphe Quetelet was trying to determine whether mathematical laws of probability could be applied to human beings. These statistical laws were commonplace in astronomy, and Quetelet believed that such laws also governed human affairs. Quetelet gathered data from French and Scottish army conscripts, including weights and heights. For each height, he found a range of weights in a normal distribution. In charting these distributions, Quetelet noticed that the weight of "normal" conscripts was proportional to their height squared. This is the general formula that would later be used to determine BMI. Since the average conscript's weight was proportional to his height, Quetelet argued that this must be what the *ideal* weight should be. A deviation from this average was considered overweight or underweight.

A century and a half later, a BMI (that is kilograms over meters squared) less than 18.5 indicates that one is underweight, a BMI beween 18.5 and 24.9 is normal, a BMI between 25 and 29.9 is overweight, a BMI between 30 and 39.9 is obese, and a BMI over 40 is morbidly obese. Quetelet's work was part of a larger wave of scientific attempts to categorize, measure, and differentiate groups in society (other techniques included measuring skulls, brows, and body proportions). Most of these efforts at measurement were meant to identify criminals or justify racial or economic discrimination. In many ways, the contemporary use of BMI fits easily with these other techniques of measurement. But Quetelet did not claim that BMI was an appropriate gauge of someone's health. In the 1940s, a statistician at Metropolitan Life Insurance Company, Louis Dublin, started charting the death rates of policy holders using a height-to-weight index. Dublin found that thinner people lived longer. He used his research to come up with ranges for each height of an "ideal" body weight. Following Dublin's lead, doctors, epidemiologists, and the federal government soon began using these tables to analyze health. The current BMI craze owes much of its popularity to the avalanche of research that followed from Dublin's work. The goal of such research is often to correlate BMI with some health problem.

Many people, however, have begun to argue that BMI is actually a poor indicator of health, and that the fad of studies demonstrating statistical correlations between BMI and specific diseases do not tell us anything about health (Oliver, 2006, pp. 21–28). In addition, the actual BMI scale with the labels "overweight," "obese," and so forth, was the product of a long, complicated decision-making process. This process relied on much more than clear, objective scientific evidence. According to Eric Oliver:

> The U.S. government's proclamation of what BMI level was overweight or obese was based, in reality, on a subjective and arbitrary call on the part of just a few researchers. Ironically, the same NIH panel that strove for "evidence-based" and objective criteria ended up making a major proclamation that, in retrospect, appears to have been for reasons that had nothing to do with health and a lot to do with the funding dynamics within the scientific professions and the pharmaceutical industry. (p. 28)

Here Oliver is referring to a report produced by the National Institutes of Health (NIH) in 1988 that concluded that the official designations of overweight should be set at a BMI of over 25 and obesity at over 30. This is still the definitive guide for determining what counts as overweight. As told by Oliver, the story of the social construction of the obesity epidemic and the ideological influences behind the development of this epidemic is clearly as much a matter of morality and politics as it is of science. But this story is made possible by the conflation of measurement and judgment that was evident from as early as Quetelet's work. In this case, it is not the conflation of measurement and judgment of food but of bodies. From this perspective, obesity is not a problem that nutrition has failed to solve or could possibly solve with the invention of new and better food guides. But rather, this is a problem that the discourse of quantification has helped invent. Because of the fervent commitment to the quantification of food and diet, it should not be surprising that quantification has become the central tool for determining health. It is within the context of the rise of this quantitative epidemic that the Food Guide Pyramid offers dietary advice. Such a context obviously blinds one to the qualitative dimensions of health. The depth, the resilience, and the ubiquity of the discourse of quantification allows the food pyramid to fit seamlessly and naturally into the social context of the moment and ensures that the constitutive features of, and qualitative judgments we make about, our foods, diets, bodies, and health are all part of a new numeric literacy.

Seeing Too Little: Crafting a New Food Guide

After the McGovern report, the USDA published a stopgap guide called "The Hassle-free guide to a better diet," in 1980. The Hassle-Free guide advised the consumption of the same number of daily servings of each food group as the 1956 Basic Four but left off the "or more" advice on the number of servings. Where the 1956 Basic Four counseled "2 *or more* 2–3 oz servings from the Meat group," the Hassle-Free diet suggested "2 servings of 2–3 oz" from the group. Also, foods that were touted as pleasurable additions to "round out meals" or to "make meals flavorful and satisfying" in 1956, were sequestered into their own group of "Fats, Sweets and Alcohol" in 1980 (Page and Phipard, 1956, p. 13). Consumption of this illicit group was "dependent on caloric needs," which highlighted the need for moderation (Welsh, 1994, p. 1800S).

The Hassle-Free guide was a temporary solution to a much larger problem. The USDA needed a new food guide to address the shift in the nutritional paradigm outlined by the *Dietary Goals*. Before crafting a new guide, the USDA and the Department of Health and Human Services collaborated to issue clear dietary guidelines that would outline lifestyle and food choice changes that consumers could expect to be quantified in the new guide.[9] The goal of these dietary guidelines for Americans was to supplement the quantitative logic of the food guide with some basic principles of healthy living. These lifestyle guidelines were no less quantitative than the food guides. The guidelines, published in 1980, made recommendations to "Eat a variety of foods; Maintain ideal weight; Avoid too much fat, saturated fat and cholesterol; Eat foods with adequate starch and fiber; Avoid too much sugar; Avoid too much sodium; and if you drink alcohol do so in moderation" (*Nutrition and Your Health*, 1980, p. 1). Because of industry pressure, the guidelines were cautious about their wording and thus "avoid too much" replaced the controversial phrase "eat less." The DHHS needed to propose lifestyle choices to combat the problem of an expanding waistline but could not offend the commercial interests of the meat, dairy, and sugar industries who lobbied the government for the syntactical change.

With the publication of these dietary guidelines in 1980, the USDA began working on a new food guide to replace the makeshift Hassle-Free guide. This new guide had to establish a diet for the new nutritional paradigm of "less is more" and had to help Americans put new dietary philosophies to use. The new food guide had to focus on the total diet rather than just the foundation of the diet, and it sought to promote "overall health." All of the food guides prior to 1980 were noted as "foundation diets," that is, the eater was supposed to follow the guide to create a good foundation of their diet and supplement it where they saw fit. The new food guide dictated all of the servings, portion sizes, and calories deemed necessary for the eater. But while the USDA could easily address the eater as a set of numbers delineated by their caloric intake or calcium requirements, they could not address the eater as an individual with particular eating preferences, favorite foods, or rituals of the table. Through their food guides the USDA systematically repressed discourses of taste that drew authority from alternative knowledge like experience, history, or geography. By ignoring these subjective elements the food guides made clear that knowing food did not involve tasting it or identifying flavors or memories or cooking techniques. Instead, knowing food involved identifying limits of calories, servings, and nutrients. For the USDA the philosophy of their new food guide was clear: numbers and quantities underpinned the basic principles that formed an epistemology of quality food.

Both the 1977 McGovern report and the 1980 dietary guidelines caused controversy among some doctors who thought that the scientific evidence underpinning some of the guidance was speculative.[10] In order to abate conflicting scientific messages and to present the information as supported by a unified scientific voice, the 1992 food guide had to "follow the same sound research process as the development of recommended levels of nutrient intake" (*USDA'S Food Guide*, 1993, p. 5). The development of the new guide was to be fully documented and open to peer review by "expert groups," and it had to reference the accepted food composition and food consumption databases to demonstrate that the goals of the guide could be achieved. The research base for the new food guide "took about 3 years to develop and document. The research was extensively peer-reviewed and use of the new daily food guide was pilot-tested before it was published for the professional community in a USDA administrative report and in a professional journal for nutrition education" (p. 7). This new guide had numerically definitive nutritional goals that employed a secondary discourse of quantification to arbitrate quality.

The new guide split the basic four into five groups by splitting fruits and vegetables into two separate groups, and removed group status from fats, sweets, and oils. Based on the nutrient content in each group, ease of use, and common eating practices, the guide could determine a proper serving size. The serving size chosen by the USDA was "a unit of measure which consumers could easily multiply or divide to represent the amount they actually eat" (p. 9). This guide was clear about the relationship between food and the American eater: food was fodder for calculation and measurement, not personal judgment.

Earlier USDA guides were largely text based. While many of the guides contained pictures of food, inclusion of the pictures was simply for context and not manifestations of the food guide's overall message. In the 1992 guide, the USDA wanted its main messages summarized in a graphic that was proportional, geometric, and, according to "graphic development research," easy for the public to remember.

> To bring the new food guide to the attention of consumers, there was need for a new, separate publication explaining the food guide and bearing an appealing illustration that would convey in a memorable way the key messages of the daily food guide—variety, proportionality, and moderation. (*USDA's Food Guide*, 1993, p. 18)

Determining what the graphic should look like was no easy task. The symbol had to be simple enough to remember and complex enough to contain all of the quantitative recommendations from the USDA. The diagram had to illustrate quantitative concepts like proportion and moderation, as well as indicate, through these quantitative concepts, "good" and "bad" foods. The new graphic had to transform the terms of quantity into a visual object and in so doing act to construct an understanding of quality. In 1988 the Human Nutrition Information Service (HNIS) hired Porter Novelli, the public relations and consumer research firm, to determine, through focus groups, a visual symbol that could communicate the "key concepts of the food guide" and "help consumers put the Dietary Guidelines into action" (*USDA's Food Guide*, 1993, p. 8). While this project's main concern is neither with the audience nor their response to the food guide, the USDA did make explicit mention of who they deemed their target audience to be. The USDA Food Guide Pyramid development document stated that their "audience was to be adults with a high school education who were not overly constrained by food cost concerns and who had eating patterns that were typical of the general U.S. population" (p. 18). The document made no mention as to what this typical eating pattern might consist of, nor did they give explicit economic standards as to what constituted an American that was not overly constrained by food costs when determining what to eat.

The USDA and Porter Novelli tested five graphic presentations among the focus groups: a circle, blocks in a row, blocks in a circle, a funnel, and a pyramid. One by one, the designs were eliminated. The circle was too familiar, and the worry was that its lack of novelty would cause its message to be ignored. While the blocks in a circle were easy to remember (it was called the 2-3-6 A Day) the focus group found the design unbalanced and "hard on the eyes." Most of the focus group disliked the funnel design because it was "unsettling and off-balance." The participants found the pyramid the most appealing. The focus group found it "easy to memorize" and the concept of proportionality, the key quantitative message of the new food guide, was evident to them. The groups closer to the base of the pyramid were the "good" foods. Because these took up a greater portion of the pyramid, they ought to constitute a greater portion of the diet. As the pyramid tapered in toward the top, the size of the groups got increasingly smaller. The base of the pyramid was breads, cereals, and grains, above them a level containing the two groups of fruits and vegetables, followed by another level containing the milk and meat groups. The very tip of the pyramid contained the groups of fats, oils, and sweets, their size indicating that their consumption should be limited. The USDA seemed proud of their design, and its ability to deliver a complex quantitative message simply:

> Overall, participants understood that the sizes of the sections of the pyramid were intended to convey the relative amounts to eat of the various food groups. [One participant stated,] "The bulk of the pyramid is things that are good for you and the little top is things you should avoid." (*USDA's Food Guide*, 1993, p. 20)

The ability of the geometric design to convey this information was a triumph of simplification for the USDA. The new graphic reduced a profusion of data, the sets of numbers and standards, and the increasingly complex and multilayered discourse of quantification into a simple figure.

The Pyramid may be a simple figure but it sought to communicate the most elaborate and sophisticated discourse of quantification to date. Each of the sections of the Pyramid also announces the number of servings per day of each food group (6–11 servings of bread and cereal, 2–3 servings of meat and fish, etc.), which established a direct relationship between a number of servings and a visual proportion of the Pyramid. The number of servings is determined by the number of calories per day one needs (for example, 1,600 for "sedentary women" or 2,800 for teenage boys). What counts as a serving must also be quantified and clarified (1 cup of yogurt or 2 ounces of processed cheese counts as a serving from the milk group). The quantities of fat, cholesterol, sugar, and salt are then listed for each food. And finally, the end of the guide offers a workbook for you to "rate your diet" (p. 28). This exercise is a perfect illustration of the capacity of the discourse of quantification to make explicit qualitative judgments. The first step in this exercise is to write down everything "you ate yesterday" and then identify the number of grams of fat in each thing (p. 28). Then one must identify how many servings one had from each group and whether or not one had had too much from any particular group. Based on these quantitative assessments, one would know what changes to make for a "healthier" diet.

By February 1991, the HNIS had the Pyramid reviewed and cleared by the USDA for publication, and a press run of a million copies was scheduled for the end of April of that year. A mere two weeks before the Pyramid was scheduled for release to the public, several newspaper articles leaked information about the food guide's new message, and its illustrated conceptualization of proportionality. On April 10, 1991, Marian Burros of the *New York Times* wrote "Rethink 4 Food Groups, Doctors Tell U.S." While this article did not mention the Food Pyramid or the USDA, it hinted at a new message to eat less meat and dairy and presented the Physicians Committee for Responsible Medicine recommended food groups: whole grains, vegetables, legumes, and fruits. Burros wrote: " 'Meat and dairy should have a much smaller place on the menu,' " said one of the committee members, Dr. Oliver Alabaster, director of the Institute for Disease Prevention at George Washington University Medical Center. 'The real point is to de-emphasize meat and dairy.' The proposed food groups 'merely dictate what would be the center of the diet,' he added" (Burros, 1991, p. C1).

Malcolm Gladwell, then at the *Washington Post*, hinted more heavily at the new Pyramid and its contents in his April 13, 1991, column, "U.S. Rethinks, Redraws the Food Groups":

> Responding to new concerns about the American diet, Agriculture Department officials have announced that they are about to replace the "food-wheel" that graced the walls of many a grade-school classroom since the 1950s with an "Eating Right Pyramid." The change puts grains and cereals at the broad base of the pyramid, fruits and vegetables on the next level, meat and dairy products in a narrow band near the top and fats and oils at the peak. The graphic device is intended to emphasize that some of the basic food groups—the big ones at the bottom of the pyramid—are more important to a healthy diet than others. (A1)

These articles incited a flurry of complaints by industry groups who were displeased with the Pyramid and its message. While the Pyramid's ability to convey proportionality elated the USDA, the National Cattlemen's Association, whose meat group was proportionally smaller than grains, fruit, and vegetables, was furious. The cattlemen, along with the National

Milk Producers Federation and the American Meat Institute, complained to Secretary of Agriculture Edward Madigan (R-IL) and demanded that he withdraw the Pyramid.

Although the previous food guide did not sell itself as a guide with a visual component, it gave the impression that meat and milk were equally as important as fruit, vegetables, and grains. In addition to the older guide's textual "eat more" message, the four food groups were visually represented as equal in size, and thus equally important in a good diet. The Pyramid's graphic illustrating proportionality became a visual epistemological basis for quality—a bigger chunk of the Pyramid meant "good" food and eat more, a smaller chunk signaled "bad" and eat less. On April 27, 1991, Madigan withdrew the Food Guide Pyramid before its public debut. According to USDA documentation, Madigan pulled the Pyramid so that it could be tested on schoolchildren and low-income adults, but articles in the press published shortly thereafter indicated that it was industry pressure to change the Pyramid's message that caused Madigan to withdraw it.

The popular press accused the USDA of bowing to lobby groups at the expense of public health. A Gladwell article in the *Washington Post* published the day the Pyramid was pulled began: "[Y]ielding to pressure from the meat and dairy industries, the Agriculture Department has abandoned its plans to turn the symbol of good nutrition from the 'food wheel' showing the 'Basic Food Groups' to an 'Eating Right' pyramid that sought to deemphasize the place of meat and dairy products in a healthy diet" (A1). A *New York Times* "Eating Well" column written by Marian Burros on May 8, 1991, entitled "Are Cattlemen Now Guarding The Henhouse?" also blamed industry pressure for the nixed Pyramid. One of that article's sources lamented the unscientific proceedings:

> Gerald Combs, who retired last Friday from the [agriculture] department as deputy administrator for human nutrition, said: "For almost eight years, until this release came out, I had had no surprises and no pressures. Issues were dealt with on the basis of scientific fact and objectivity. I was terribly upset by this announcement. I don't know of any valid reason for the decision made so abruptly and handled so badly. One can only jump to all sorts of conclusions. My concern is that people will think the department has no integrity or objectivity." (C1)

At this point, the USDA hired another market research group, Bell Associates Inc., to gather information from focus groups from low-income families and children. The USDA also assembled three additional focus groups: secondary school teachers of science and home economics, representatives of several professional associations and advocacy groups, and "food industry representatives associated with various commodity groups" (*USDA's Food Guide*, 1993, p. 24). The USDA was still concerned about proportionality, but it also became concerned with the food guide message not contain any "misinformation" (p. 23). The USDA called up a whole new set of designs as alternatives to the Food Pyramid: quarter circles and right triangles, pie charts, grocery carts, bowls, building blocks, and bar graphs. Of the alternatives, the bowl design received the most attention, and it was selected to compete with the pyramid design for the icon that most effectively delivered the information. Interestingly enough, the bowl design (with vertical divisions for each food group) did not convey the message of proportionality as well as any of the other designs—the food groups had different sized divisions, but there was no horizontal hierarchy. Regarding the bowl design the USDA report stated:

> Although the food industry group did not think it conveyed proportionality well, they liked the vertically divided bowl because it did not "stack" foods. Among all of the focus groups, however, the pyramid fared better than the bowl at communicating proportionality and moderation. Certain foods were more important in a daily diet than others, and the food pyramid best illustrated that concept. (p. 23)[11]

The reason the food industry had such disdain for the pyramid was not because of its actual shape. Had the meat group been lower in the pyramid and occupied a proportionally larger chunk, the industry dissent presumably would have been quieter. The objection to the pyramid came from its visual hierarchy, and the ability of the illustration to spatially rank the quality of a food. In a bowl shape, all of the food groups were equally close to the foundation. In the pyramid, certain groups were several steps away from the all-important pyramid base. The illustration that the USDA was going to use to represent the new nutritional message was not only important in that it had to represent a discourse, but it also had to spatially represent good and bad. In the diagram, the USDA wanted readers to see quality. After a year of research, and nearly 1 million dollars later, the USDA rereleased the Food Guide Pyramid. While the focus groups preferred the design of the bowl by a small margin, it was mainly because they associated a bowl with food. In illustrating concepts of proportionality and moderation, the pyramid remained the preferred design. On April 28, 1992, USDA Secretary Madigan released the Food Guide Pyramid, and aside from changing a few of the food pictures (elbow macaroni to spaghetti; a milk carton to a glass of milk), the pyramid remained the same.

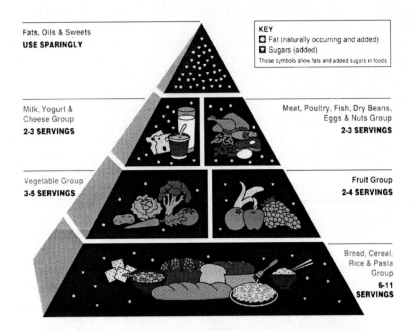

Figure 2. USDA Food Guide Pyramid, 1992. From "The Food Guide Pyramid," *USDA Home and Garden Bulletin*, no. 252. (Source: USDA)

The Rhetorical Effects of the Pyramid

The process of selecting a graphic, and the political ramifications and message the graphic represented, illustrates the rhetorical capacity of images to refigure our understanding of everyday objects. Richard Buchanan (2001) treats design as a rhetorical tool, and sees design as "reuniting things and words—*res et verba*" (p. 185). The Food Guide Pyramid was an attempt to bring together a discourse and a picture, and thus the way the USDA portrayed that discourse in order to maintain rhetorical fidelity was important. Buchanan argues, "In essence, design offers a pathway for bringing theory—ideas about the nature of the world and how we should live our lives—into closer relationship with practical action and the creation of diverse kinds of products and experiences" (p. 186). The goal of the design of the Food Guide Pyramid was twofold. First, it had to illustrate the "ideas about the nature of the world" that is, quantitative concepts like proportionality and moderation. These theoretical ideas were distilled from the scientific tradition and the quantitative discourse that informed the USDA nutrition policy. Second, the pyramid design had to inform us "how we should live our lives." The pyramid had to suggest courses of action and encourage us to experience food in a particular way. Much of the fuss around the design of the pyramid pointed to the incommensurability between the courses of action that the food industry wanted to recommend, and those courses of action that the USDA wanted to recommend.

Because the Food Guide Pyramid had to illustrate the shift from "more" to "less," Buchanan's "theory" collided with "practical action" in a controversial way. Buchanan also puts this diagrammatic unification of theory and practice in a different way:

> One of the commonplaces that remain with us as a legacy of the Renaissance is the distinction between the fine and useful arts. The fine arts were associated with the liberal arts and mathematics, usually representing a vision of the Platonic ideal. In contrast, the useful arts were regarded as servile, materialistic, and lacking the degree of thought that belongs to mathematics and the liberal and fine arts. (p. 186)

This distinction is illustrated in the USDA's concern that the pyramid should be "easy to remember." The USDA wanted the message of the new guide to be simple and accessible to all audiences. By manifesting the new nutritional message in an icon, the USDA codified the rhetorical role of a discourse of quantification. The USDA saw the pyramid as a functioning technology that took the language of a discipline and made it more common in a picture. The Food Guide Pyramid illustrated quantities, connoted qualities, and encouraged Americans to adopt a new understanding of what kind of food they should eat.

The USDA's visual component to their new nutritional message was an important rhetorical tool for several other reasons as well. First, the new graphic representation of a discourse of quantification represented a moment of its reification. The terms of science, and the groups of numbers that had come to define nutrition guidance in the past, now had a referent: a simple symbol that could stand in for an increasingly complex and confusing language. In *The Rhetoric of Science*, Alan Gross (1996) addresses the reifying ability of a visual sign as playing an important role in construction and acceptance of a scientific argument: "By means of normalization . . . figures perform a crucial ontological role in the transformation of the terms of science into theoretically important physical objects and events" (p. 75). A discourse of quantification, and its constant definition and redefinition of good and bad through its terms of more and less, is transformed with the Food Pyramid into a real object. By transforming quantitative terms into physical objects, and in reifying a discourse of quantification, the food guide concurrently reinforced the authoritative role of science as the arbiter of quality.

Second, while the new visual acted to codify a discourse of quantification and make visible the now quantitative nature of quality, it also secured the stronghold of this discourse as the sole language for addressing the American eater. Scott Montgomery (1996) explains the ability of a visual representation to abrogate other forms of knowledge or organizing principles:

> Considering the stories of how terms and images in science have arisen can demonstrate how distinctly nontechnical, and at times highly emotional and political, concepts have come to be codified as organizing principles within the very heart of scientific thought—to the extent of furthering certain possibilities for knowing the world at the expense of others. (p. 138)

Once a discourse of quantification became visible through the graphic representation of the pyramid, this image could negate other discourses of quality because it had, in its corner, an external referent. It was this palpability that made it difficult for alternative discourses to carve out spaces for themselves, or to compete with a discourse of quantification. Gross (1996) argues that tables and figures join with the text to shape judgment, and "to mobilize all the means of persuasion in the interest of a particular cause. By raising the price of dissent, tables and figures work together with text to win scientific arguments" (p. 80).

If the pyramid, as a rhetorical tool, represents the transformation of a scientific and numeric discourse into a seeable icon that attempts to persuade its audience to eat, and by extension understand, food in a particular, enumerated way, then how does it do this? How does a figure help win an argument? Answering this question requires that we read the pyramid as a rhetorical trope. *Trope* literally means "to turn," and, clearly, the Food Pyramid is designed to turn our attention from one aspect of food to another. In this case, the Pyramid works by turning the public's attention toward numeric calculation and away from any other aspect of food (its taste, seasonality, etc.). In other words, the Pyramid is designed to represent a mathematical formula (even though that is not the ordinary signification of a pyramid), and thus it certifies that the real nature of food is found in its numeric properties. When Gross (1996) claims that "figures perform a crucial ontological role in the transformation of the terms of science into theoretically important physical objects and events," he is partly right (p. 75). To extend his claim, tropes and figures can reinscribe, on physical objects and events, a new kind of being. The Pyramid refigures food by making its numeric properties the only reality worth representing.

For example, all of the pictures of food in the 1992 guide are abstract and cartoonish, not literal. These pictures of foods, therefore, are representations of representations and thus serve only to further certify numeric realities. To have a literal picture of cheese, chicken, or grapes would risk creating other kinds of associations with other discourses. Whether these pictures are read in a polysemous manner is beside the point. The use of abstract representations attempts to legitimate quantitative evaluations and neglect or override qualitative evaluations. Once the assumption that numbers constitute the real properties of food is in place, the discourse of quantification controls epistemological claims and the task of judgment. In addition to certifying a particular ontological conception of food, the figure or trope of the pyramid is designed to simplify matters of knowing and judging. The Food Pyramid also illustrates how numbers work as tropes. Numbers, as I have shown throughout, are the linguistic means by which foods are refigured in nutrition guides. On their surface, these numbers signify an abstract quantity, the interpretation of which is not a matter of open debate or disagreement. But to trope is to employ words in such a way that one's attention is turned from one thing to another. From a rhetorical perspective, numbers act just like other words. In this case, numbers, quantities, and statistics trope food groups by turning one's attention to the chemical composition of foods and away from the possibilities of pleasure. These numbers also turn one's attention from the language games provided by one's cultural experiences of eating to a discourse of quantification.

The Food Pyramid and its quantitative dietary advice, however, was not the only way of thinking about eating and health in this period. What Warren Belasco has called the "countercuisine" offered a "coherent set of dietary beliefs and practices" (1993, p. 4). This countercuisine suggested that consumers avoid processed foods and believed that improvisation, craftsmanship, and regional cooking could make food fun. The countercuisine also promoted the development of communal farms and cooperative groceries. The government officials and scientists that advocated for the food pyramid generally opposed the organic movement and the radical suggestions for revolutionizing farming methods. The mainstream food establishment also remained ambivalent about fear of processed foods and additives.

The countercuisine made nutritional arguments about the difference between natural and plastic foods. Natural foods, from this perspective, were

safer and tastier, and vegetarianism, often a core belief of the countercuisine, seemed both ecologically and spiritually sound, and organic gardening
was a path to self-discovery and social protest. The oppositional identity
crafted by this movement found joy and health by contrasting their own
foods, preparation techniques, dining etiquette, and health recommendations with the mainstream scientists and government officials crafting and
promoting the Food Guide Pyramid. The nutrition mainstream eventually
tried to distinguish between what was considered healthy from the other
fads, or extreme and foolish suggestions, advocated by the countercuisine.
Throughout the 1980s the organic paradigm questioned and challenged
conventional science and agribusiness, causing some significant changes.
But the mainstream approach to science and government-sponsored dietary
advice, along with its ideological commitment to quantification, managed
to continue to control the common sense view of food and eating. The
countercuisine remained at the fringes of the debate. This was not inevitable, but the alignment of science, government, and industry proved too
effective at dispensing dietary advice.

Another Way to See the Pyramid

This story of the origins of the food pyramid makes three contributions to
an understanding of the rhetoric of science. First, rhetorics of science are
not only capable of inventing objects like quarks and double helices, such
rhetorics also have the potential to remake the objects of our everyday
use. When Gross (1996) redescribes discovery as "invention" he attempts
to capture, through rhetorical analysis, how science is a generative enter-
prise (p. 7). But science is also, at times, a project of redescription or
reinvention—this is exactly what happens in the case of American food
guidance—the foods we eat are refigured by language. Second, examining
a food guide without examining the development of the language of the
guide over time would be to perform rhetorical criticism in a vacuum.
Rhetorics of science must account for the historical ways that scientific
languages develop and the cumulative effects of those languages. All histories of science are also rhetorical histories. Third, images or symbols
naturalize and certify realities that otherwise might be contested. Scientific
images represent a world that we come to assume is given, but in fact
those images make up that given world.

From a public health perspective, a rhetorical history of food guides
illustrates that future public health policy will always be a matter of numeric
evaluation, so long as the discourse of quantification is the controlling
discourse. In order to secure public health one must know how to count,

and make evaluations of quality based on what one counted. The question becomes: does the use of a discourse of quantification *really* improve public health? It is certainly clear that this discourse shifts and changes to meet whatever social exigence exists in a given context. But in doing so, health is refigured as well. "Eating healthy" is a moving target. How does one improve a moving target? The answer to this question is not clear, but it must be found in the rhetorical imagination and rhetorical practice of those engaged in figuring public health.

Dissent then, just as it was costly for any external body to introduce an alternative epistemology of quality of food, was also costly for the USDA. When the social exigency of corpulence presented itself, the USDA responded by further concretizing their discourse of quantification, and by using it to define and solve the problem at hand. When they were faced with a new nutritional problem, the USDA did not reevaluate their framework for understanding food. Instead, they reaffirmed their faith in the discourse that they had always used by rendering it concrete. The Food Pyramid itself simply moved around food groups, created physical representations of sets of numbers, and recast the quantitative concept of proportionality. The Food Pyramid did not reevaluate the notion of using numbers to order and organize the relationship between Americans and food. However, as we will see in the next chapter, alternatives to the Pyramid do not question or change the methods used or assumptions made by a discourse of quantification. Instead, they work within, and perpetuate, the framework already established by the USDA, and they too rely on the language and symbols of science.

The Food Pyramid ensnares its readers by making numbers more real than the objects those numbers originally represented. Thus judgment is only possible within the discursive framework provided and perpetuated by the entire history of American food guidance and nutrition policy. In the latest step in this history, on April 19, 2005, the secretary of the United States Department of Agriculture released a new and improved Food Guide Pyramid. This pyramid, called MyPyramid, was supposed to represent "Steps to a Healthier You," and aimed to provide, the new "best" daily food choices for Americans. Lines radiate from the pyramid's apex, creating different colored and sized wedges. Each colored wedge represents a food group and the proportion of each food group that the "healthier you" should eat. For example, the largest wedge is the orange-colored grains group, the group that healthy Americans should consume most often. A tiny yellow sliver of the pyramid, is a group named oils, a group that is "needed for health" but whose intake "needs to be limited" to "balance total calorie intake." Just as with the first pyramid, every group is sized according to how much of each group one should eat. This new pyramid has three dimensions and a set of steps up the side. A stick figure is rendered running up the side of the pyramid. This figure is to represent the *"moderate* or *vigorous"* physical activity that Americans should engage in for "at least 30 minutes per day." In figuring the healthy national diet in such a way, the USDA continues to rely on the public's understanding of proportionality, quantities, and sanctioned serving sizes of foods. This new pyramid is yet another example of rhetorical imagination and rhetorical practice used in the service of a discourse of quantification.

Perhaps the most unique characteristic of this new guide is the MyPyramid tracker. This tracker allows users to enter their weight, age, and everything that they have eaten over the course of a number of days. The tracker then analyzes the quality of your diet and determines the amount by which you are either exceeding or falling short of the recommended intake of specific food groups. Here the mathematical calculation of health is done by the software on the website for each user. The tracker even allows the user a series of choices for each food he selects to determine what he considers a serving size. For example, if you were to enter in "cheese pizza," you would then be expected to determine the size of the pizza (measured in inches in diameter). Then the dietary guidelines appear on the screen with small emoticons representing happy faces, sad faces, and neutral faces to tell the user what nutritional categories had been satisfied for the day, ignored, or exceeded. In this manner, one could track one's daily caloric intake, break that caloric intake down in terms of one's particular nutritional needs, and then the software will recommend dietary changes to either improve health or lose weight. One portion of pizza, for example, exceeds the number of fat grams recommended for the day. The dietary advice is simple in such a case—stop eating cheese pizza. This is another example of a technology of governance that can inscribe a sense of ethical incompleteness on the user. Perhaps more importantly, it reduces the user's health strictly to a numerical evaluation. From the perspective of the USDA, the effectiveness of software like the MyPyramid tracker is in its numerical accuracy. The same value that guided Atwater's early experiments in calorimetry guides the invention of internet software like the MyPyramid tracker. Pizza is nothing more than the proportion of calories and nutrients within my recommended daily diet. And my health is a matter of whether or not I exceed those recommendations.

The latest numerical standard invented by the USDA makes this last argument clear—the Healthy Eating Index. The Healthy Eating Index is a measure of diet quality that assesses conformance to federal dietary guidance. It was created by the USDA in 1995 and revised in 2005 to be used along with MyPyramid. The index includes a set of scoring standards—points awarded for the consumption of particular foods. One's diet is scored using this point system (the average score in the United States was 63.8), and one's health is judged based on the range within which the score falls. The Healthy Eating Index is a complete triumph for the discourse of quantification and the reduction of health to the confines of this discourse. It is also an indication of the erosion of culture, tradition, experience, and taste in the social practice of eating. At least it seems that the U.S. government has been, and continues to be, deeply invested in the eradication of such factors in our choices of what to eat. The history of the development of the Food Guide Pyramid makes that clear.

Chapter Four

Scaling the Pyramid

Criticisms of the USDA

The USDA Food Guide Pyramid had a very clear message: "limit fat to 30% of calories."[1] Obesity, type 2 diabetes, and heart disease were on the rise (and had been since before the 1977 McGovern report), and the USDA claimed that fat was the primary cause of these problems. One of the Pyramid's goals, then, was to educate consumers about the perils of fat in their diet. Since the USDA didn't want America to eat fat, it encouraged them to consume starch in its place. Because starches were relatively fat-free, the logic was that by reducing the calorie-dense fat in the diet and replacing it with starches that had comparatively fewer calories per gram, America's obesity problem would begin to subside and rates of diabetes and heart disease would decline. This was not the case. American obesity rates and deaths from diet-attributed heart attacks continued to rise. By the mid to late 1990s some critics sensed a causal link between the USDA's nutrition messages and diet related health problems. Obesity and its associated health problems had become an epidemic, and the first place critics looked for explanations was the USDA Food Guide Pyramid. America seemed to be heeding USDA advice to eat less fat, but their overall caloric intake was increasing.[2] Eating from the wide swath of low-fat starch at the pyramid base, the "good" foods, was not creating a healthy public.

Obesity is, of course, the paradigmatic disease of quantification, and the political and social choices that have shaped the invention of the standards for obesity have relied on "fat science" for justification. But as a disease, "obesity is a flawed construct" (Oliver, 2006, p. 37) because it is not "an interruption, cessation, or disorder of body function, system, or organ," as *Stedman's Medical Dictionary* defines disease. If obesity is not a classic instance of disease, why, then, did it become an epidemic? Moreover, why did this new epidemic drive critiques of the Food Guide Pyramid? In 1997 William Dietz became director of the Division for Nutrition and Physical Activity at the Centers for Disease Control and Prevention. Dietz held the view that obesity was influenced by the environment, and was something that happened to people. This allowed him to think of obesity as a disease. In order to convince the public that this was the case, Dietz used years of statistical data from annual telephone surveys of health patterns in the United States to show changing rates of obesity over the last 15 years. In 1998 he began presenting this data as a series of maps. These maps presented a frightening picture of recent weight gains. On each slide, a map of the United States was shown with different colors to signify different rates of obesity in a given year. The presentation was able to show the development, progress, and growth of these rates from year to year, and the growth appeared to be dramatic, as if it were a spreading infection. Despite being misleading in several important ways (for example, using the geographic size of a state as a stand-in for population size), these maps were very effective in generating significant concern about this growing "epidemic." Most importantly, these maps are illustrative of the use of a discourse of quantification in the invention of a disease. It was in this context that critics of the Food Guide Pyramid tried to craft improved quantitative advice.

But critics of the Food Guide Pyramid had neither the same ethos nor the same means for disseminating their nutritional message as the USDA. Thus, critics of the Pyramid relied on media outlets to publicize their alternatives to the federal nutrition agenda. These alternatives appeared on television shows such as the *Today* show and *60 Minutes*, in national broadsheet publications like the *Washington Post*, the *New York Times*, and the *Wall Street Journal*, in several national news magazines, and on radio broadcasts. Media coverage lent credence to the criticisms, helped in their publicity, and helped to craft them as viable alternatives.

In this chapter, I examine three critiques, or pyramid alternatives, that received ample coverage in the popular press. While other alternatives existed, many were iterations of the three main criticisms highlighted in this chapter. What is most important, however, is that while each alternative presented itself as both different and better than the USDA Food Guide Pyramid, each alternative demonstrated the extent to which a discourse of quantification reigned as the default manner to discuss food. Thus, criticisms about federal nutrition were made using a language of measurements, numbers, and science. Valid criticisms called into question the USDA's numbers but did not call into question the use of a discourse of quantification itself. Criticisms that lay at the discursive level of culture or taste could be dismissed as too subjective or unscientific.[3] The power of numbers to determine valid arguments, and the influence of the topos of quantity, meant that in order to challenge the USDA, critics had to use the same language. The best available means for articulating problems of the American diet was a discourse of quantification, and the only way to solve those problems was expanding and building on the language of numbers.

Therefore, in the face of the USDA Pyramid, critics began to produce more numbers: measurements of success and failure rates of the Pyramid, measurements of portion size, serving size and American appetites, and measurements of "good" and "bad" micro-nutrients in "good" and "bad" food and drink. With growing numbers of criticisms, the conflation of measurement and judgment became increasingly bound up with discussions of portion control and meal choice. Each critique further established the power of a discourse of quantification to control both knowledge about food and eating practices. Because the critiques relied on science, each illustrated the authority of the scientific voice and its ability to both invent and solve its own problems. By inventing additional vocabularies, symbols, and words, the discourse of quantification continued to expand and extend its influence, becoming more self-referential along the way. Numbers established as intrinsic qualities of food now referred to other numbers thus reinforcing their own viability and importance. The expansion of a discourse of quantification was abetted by USDA critics who used the USDA's own numeric discursive framework to criticize. By virtue of their attention to science, the critics of the Food Guide Pyramid also demonstrated how their own relationship to food was ordered and controlled by the historical supremacy of this discourse of quantification. The critic's work is judged by the ability to accurately and objectively measure the shortcomings of the Food Guide Pyramid and correct those shortcomings with an appropriately refined language shaped by new calculations and quantities. Critiques of the Pyramid fault it for irresponsible numeration but propose a solution to this irresponsibility with more numbers.

The first critique of the USDA Pyramid arises from within U.S. federal agencies. According to this critique a major problem with the Food Guide Pyramid and its application in everyday life is that while it relied on a number of servings of certain foods per day, the quantitative concept of the "serving" was not standardized. The problem, then, was that Americans were confused and did not know what "how much" was. In other words, inadequate consumer information was the root of the problem.

This critique advocates more education about what quantity constitutes a serving as compared to a portion and it advocates the standardization of a proper portion size. The former is a USDA quantity and the latter is what the eater actually consumes.

The second critique manifests itself in an alternative eating plan to the one proposed by the Food Guide Pyramid. This alternative recognizes an epistemology of quality founded in quantitative terms, but charges the USDA with attaching incorrect quantities to notions of quality. The most noteworthy of these critics is Walter Willett, the chairman of the Department of Nutrition at the Harvard School of Public Health, and a professor of medicine at Harvard Medical School. Willett contends that the Food Guide Pyramid treats carbohydrates and fats as absolutely "good" and "bad," a categorization that is faulty, based on outdated science, and is a danger to public health. Willett's remedy for the Pyramid's misclassification of good and bad is to reclassify these categories by adding new numeric criteria for judging quality. Not all carbohydrates are good according to his critique, only those that have a low glycemic index number and a high fiber content. Conversely, according to Willett's alternative, not all fats are bad. This critique reclassifies fats that are derived from plant sources and unsaturated as good. These fats are even better if they provide a measurable source of alpha-linoleic acid or Omega-3 fatty acids. Willett's criticism recognizes that defining quality food relies on quantities, and does not challenge that epistemology.

A third proposed alternative to the USDA's Food Guide Pyramid is the emergence of the French Paradox and the Mediterranean Diet as a cultural "lifestyle" of dietary habits. The Mediterranean Diet uses data from a series of population studies in France, Italy, and Greece that link the low incidence of coronary heart disease to the consumption of olive oil and red wine—ingredients that are local to the region and traditional to Mediterranean cultures. The Oldways Preservation and Exchange Trust and the World Health Organization proposed this "cultural model of healthy eating" to replace the USDA's Food Guide Pyramid. Because this critique employs a cultural framework to encourage certain patterns of eating, it hints at a divergence from a discourse of quantification. This proposal for a new diet, however, is a return to the commonplace of quantity. Arguments for the Mediterranean Diet rely on public health population statistics and scientific analyses of the chemical components of wine as their persuasive tools. In regard to this critique, I examine the discourse of quantification around red wine, a controversial component of the Mediterranean Diet. Proponents of the Mediterranean Diet crafted an alternative to the Food Guide Pyramid by abstracting and measuring the diet of Mediterranean cultures, and, in particular, the frequency and volume of their red wine consumption. By stripping away all cultural aspects of wine and quantifying the "goodness" of red wine, the cultures of the Mediterranean became something that could be prescribed, dosed, and controlled in the American diet.

The criticisms of the Food Guide Pyramid, and the proposed alternatives for "how to eat," point to the extent to which a discourse of quantification directs both policy and public health initiatives regarding food in America. Discourses that address taste, pleasure, or the social significance of food are absent from proposals that encourage Americans to eat well, and they repeat discursive patterns established by the USDA. While all of the critiques employ different arguments, none criticize the underlying epistemology firmly rooted in numbers, objectivity, and standards. The language for ordering and directing eating habits for the last hundred years also ordered and directed the possible responses to, and critiques of, that language.

How Much Are You Being Served?
Quantifying "Servings" and Eating "Portions"

The Food Guide Pyramid, although devoted to a rigorous and exact description of quantities, defines the daily diet in terms of servings, an imprecise and inconsistently defined quantity. Thus, the first major critique of the Food Guide Pyramid charges the USDA with confusing the American public. Exactly what constituted a serving also proved to be a source of confusion and uncertainty for the USDA. When they attempted to rectify the situation, the USDA fell back on a discourse of quantification. This demonstrated the inability of the U.S. government to discuss food as anything but a countable comestible and demonstrated the stronghold of a discourse of quantification in federal nutrition policy.[4]

As the USDA celebrated the ability of the pyramid to deliver the message of meal proportionality to the public, the Food Guide Pyramid also made explicit the number of servings per day from each food group Americans should eat. At the base of the pyramid, Americans needed 6-11 servings of bread, rice, cereal, grains, and pasta. One level up from the broad base were 3-5 servings of vegetables and 2-4 servings of fruit. The last numerically quantified level above the fruits and vegetables were the meat and milk groups, which suggested 2-3 servings per day. The USDA left the tip of the pyramid—fats, oils, and sweets—unnumerated, and counseled the eater to "use sparingly," leaving the quantitative judgment of "sparingly" up to each individual. The guide provided a range of numbers of servings for each food group. To determine how much of each group one ought to be eating, the eater had to categorize herself. The guide encouraged the eater to determine "How many servings are right for me?" Choosing what was "right," however, required little personal input. The correct number of servings per day was based on daily caloric intakes suggested by the National Academy of Sciences food consumption surveys ("Pyramid," 1992, p. 8).

The 1992 guide treated populations in a similar fashion to Wilbur Atwater's population studies 90 years earlier. But while Atwater determined caloric groups for occupations, sexes, races, and locations, the modern guide was considerably less specific. The Food Guide Pyramid only grouped Americans into three caloric categories: 1,600 calories per day (sedentary women, and older adults), 2,200 calories per day (children, teenage girls, active women, and sedentary men) and 2,800 calories per day (teenage boys, active men, and some very active women) (p. 8). These caloric groups determined the number of servings of each food group one ought to eat.

> [I]f you are an active woman who needs about 2,200 calories a day, 9 servings of breads, cereals and rice, or pasta would be right for you. You'd also want to eat about 6 ounces of meat or alternates per day. Keep total fat (fat in the foods you choose as well as fat used in cooking or added at the table) to about 73 grams per day. (p. 9)

In attempting to answer the individual and idiosyncratic question "How many servings are right for me?," the USDA generated three general, abstract types or categories within which individuals must fit. The invention of these categories facilitated the management and control of the American eating public and eliminated personal, social, and cultural differences among eaters. The three caloric categories also created an equation for each eater, reifying the mathematics behind the pyramid.

Because the USDA had specified daily quantities of servings, they needed to provide exact measurements for what constituted each "serving." The Food Guide Pyramid booklet gives examples of servings for each of the Pyramid food groups throughout. A serving from the starch-based group is "1 slice of bread, 1 ounce of ready-to-eat cereal, or 1 cup of cooked cereal, rice, or pasta." From the "Meat, Poultry, Fish, Dry Beans, Eggs, and Nuts" group a serving is more difficult to measure, and so the Pyramid states that its recommended 2–3 servings should be the equivalent to 5–7 ounces of cooked meat per day:

Counting to see if you have an equivalent of 5–7 ounces of cooked lean meat a day is tricky. Portion sizes vary with the type of food and the meal. For example, 6 ounces might come from: 1 egg (count as 1oz of lean meat) for breakfast—2 oz of sliced turkey in a sandwich for lunch; and—3 oz cooked lean hamburger for dinner. ("Pyramid," 1992, p. 22)[5]

In order to follow the Food Guide Pyramid, eaters had to quantify themselves based on their caloric requirements, then use that categorization to measure the number of servings per day they needed. The invention of the "serving" by the USDA was important in organizing and ordering the relationship between the eater and his or her food. It served as the quantitative epistemological foundation of food choice and control. Just as the calorie had become an intrinsic numeric quality of food, the serving gave volumes of food certain quantitative qualities. In addition to choosing a food based on its numeric nutritional value, one could use the serving to guide how much of each food to eat.

Concurrent with the USDA's release of the Food Guide Pyramid, the Food and Drug Administration passed the Nutrition Labeling and Education Act (NLEA), which required all packaged foods labeled on or after May 8, 1994, to be printed with nutrition facts. The Nutrition Facts label is a small, rectangular information panel, of specific dimensions, that indicates the serving size, servings per container, calories, calories from fat, total fat, saturated fat, cholesterol, sodium, carbohydrate, sugar, fiber, and protein content of the food contained in the package. The FDA also asked that in addition to packaged foods in stores, retailers provide voluntary nutrition information for the 20 most frequently consumed fruits, vegetables, fish, and the 45 most popular cuts of meat. The Nutrition Facts label gave the eater numeric insight into what was in their box of cereal and reinforced the displacement of the concept of quality with quantity. At a glance, the eater could assess the quality of the food by consulting the facts label and determining whether the data rendered that food good or bad. The FDA hoped that the Nutrition Facts label would allow for quick comparisons of food in the grocery store and would develop numeric standards that allowed the food industry to make certain health claims.[6]

Although two separate government bodies now maintained jurisdiction over certain types of nutrition information, the goals of both the Food and Drug Administration's legislation of the NLEA and the USDA's release of the Food Guide Pyramid were the same: to create a better diet for Americans. With respect to the NLEA, the FDA declared: "one of the primary purposes of the 1990 [NLEA] amendments was to educate consumers about healthful dietary practices."[7] The Food Guide Pyramid stated that it was "an outline of what to eat each day . . . a general guide that lets you choose a healthful diet that's right for you" ("Pyramid," 1992, p. 2). Each government body had a set of numeric guidelines that aided the consumer in making what they considered to be good food choices. Many of these standards were the same: for example, the quantitative understanding of a "good" food meant that it contained less fat, less salt, and no cholesterol. But there was a quantitative inconsistency between the messages of the FDA and the USDA. There was no numeric consensus as to what quantity constituted a "serving." Thus, while Americans could try to follow the numbers in the USDA-governed Pyramid, their FDA-ruled grocery store purchases could undermine their mathematics.

Some differences between serving sizes were naught or negligible. Both the USDA and the FDA defined a slice of regular bread as a serving. Other servings were radically different—the USDA defined a serving of cooked pasta as a half a cup and the FDA's Nutrition Facts label defined a serving of the same cooked pasta as one cup. Pancakes seemed to bring even greater confusion; one serving of pancakes according to the USDA was one 4-inch pancake weighing in at 1.5 ounces and tallying 50 calories. The FDA's portion of pancakes was three 5-inch pancakes weighing 7.5 ounces and 250 calories—five times the size of the USDA serving ("Serving Sizes," 2000). Because a discourse of quantification relied on precise objective measurements for well-defined entities, this discrepancy between the servings for the USDA and the FDA undermined the rhetorical effect of the concept of a serving and rendered the discourse of quantification impotent.

The problem with defining a serving demonstrates the fundamental role language plays in shaping our knowledge of, and beliefs about, food. Critics of the Pyramid may have argued over the numbers used to define a serving but such arguments served strictly linguistic ends. While the FDA and the USDA sought to clarify the meaning of a serving, this was not a quantity that had an external referent. Unlike the calorie, a serving was not a term invented by science and applied to food. Thus, the agencies had the ability to craft a definition of the serving to serve their own ends. In so doing the USDA and FDA engaged explicitly in an act of linguistic invention that incorporated numbers and measurements. The agencies, by virtue of their arguments over the meaning of a serving, point to the importance of language in general and the necessity of fashioning a language that avails itself to desired ends. In essence this is an example of the government agencies working as rhetoricians and not policy-makers or scientists.

The quantitative measure of a serving for either agency was an arbitrary invention. The USDA Center for Nutrition Policy and Promotion defined the Food Guide Pyramid serving as "a unit of measure used to describe the total amount of foods recommended daily from each of the food groups. . . . Larger portions count as more than one serving; smaller portions count as partial servings" ("Food Portions," 1999). The USDA had four explicit factors in determining a serving size: typical portion size (which they derived from food consumption surveys), ease of use, nutrient content, and "tradition," which, for the USDA, meant referencing past food guides. According to the USDA, a typical portion size was a ½ cup of vegetables, and a traditional serving size of bread was one 2.5-ounce slice. The FDA's serving was defined as "a specific amount of food that contains the quantity of nutrients listed on the Nutrition Facts Label. . . . To make foods consumer-friendly, the serving sizes are expressed in household measures, such as cups, ounces, or pieces, as well as grams, and generally reflect the amount an individual might reasonably consume each eating occasion" ("Food Portions," 1999). The FDA criteria for a serving size were "*based on*—but not necessarily *equal to*—the amount of food customarily eaten at one time [called the "reference amount"] as reported from nationwide food consumption surveys" ("Serving Sizes," 2000, italics FDA).[8] Using terms like "reasonably," shows that the FDA, while they attempted to define a quantity, could not excise the human, subjective component of eating. Attempting to use the standard of "reasonable consumption," when crafting a quantitative definition, normalizes the entire eating population.

While the USDA uses the word "tradition" and the FDA uses the notion of "custom" and refers to an "eating occasion," both attempt to employ a discourse of quantification to define words that refer to social and cultural practices. Using these words, the USDA unwittingly evokes cultural habits that refer to an eater's relationship to food grounded on an entirely qualitative set of interests. Traditions, customs, and occasions that guide eating behavior cannot be quantified, they are part of cultural eating practices guided by an immeasurable "how" of food and not "how much."[9] By employing these terms, the USDA strips subjectivity from the eater and the eating experience, and makes tradition, custom, and occasion reference points for a quantitative epistemology of food.

The fact that the USDA attempted to quantify such historically and socially situated concepts is not a surprise. What was surprising, however, was that the criticisms of such attempts only refer to the imprecision and ambiguity of those terms and not the use of the terms themselves. The critics called on the USDA for better accuracy regarding the concept of a serving but ignored subjective aspects of culture, custom, and tradition in crafting definitions. This is a testament to the persuasive effect of a discourse of quantification. The USDA saw the *lack* of numeration as the problem, not the irreconcilability of the subjectivity of culture and the objectivity of quantity.

Instead of investigating qualitative notions of custom and tradition, the FDA and the USDA began to study how American diets were measuring up to federal standards using federally quantified terms. The USDA's Center for Nutrition Policy and Promotion developed a scoring system (the Healthy Eating Index or HEI) to rate the quality of the eater based on their food serving choices. A system of points was allotted to eaters who followed the serving guidelines of the Pyramid.

The HEI examines dietary intake in relation to servings of the five major groups in the Food Guide Pyramid: grains, vegetables, fruits, milk, and meat. The recommended number of servings depends on a person's caloric requirement:

> A maximum score of 10 was assigned to each of the five food group components of the Index if a person's diet met or exceeded the recommended number of servings for a food group. For example, if a person's diet met the fruits group serving recommendations, then that person's diet was awarded 10 points. (*Healthy Eating*, 1996)

The Healthy Eating Index data for the years 1994–1996 revealed that 88% of the U.S. population had a diet that was either "poor," with an HEI score of less than 51 points, or "needing improvement," with an HEI score of 51–80 points. When the USDA pointed out the problem of the poor diet, it defined this problem in terms of the serving:

> For most food groups, the food supply data show a substantial gap between the quantity and type of foods provided by the food supply and Food Guide Pyramid recommendations. When measured in servings, average supplies of fruits and vegetables were well below those needed to provide most Americans with the five to nine daily servings recommended by the Food Guide Pyramid. (Kantor, 1996, p. 3)

After quantifying a new aspect of the daily diet the USDA used that quantity to measure the quality of the American diet, and by extension, their success. Unfortunately, for the USDA, their "serving" was failing them, and they had the numbers to prove it.

In response to this failure, the USDA continued to generate data sets indicating "the percentage change needed to meet Food Guide Pyramid serving recommendations." According to that data set, Americans needed to increase their intake of fruit servings by 100%, increase their vegetable servings by 30% and decrease their added sugars by 70%. These pages of numbers, demographics, and statistics continued to provide the government agencies with information about what America didn't know about food. The data indicated that there was an inconsistency between the amount that Americans were eating and the amount the USDA wanted them to eat. The federal government's solution to this problem of substandard American eaters was to quantify their eating behavior so that they could better understand why Americans didn't understand. To do this, the USDA introduced another new quantitative term for food: the "portion." The portion was quite different from the serving: "A 'portion' can be thought of as the amount of a specific food an individual eats for dinner, snack, or other eating occasion. Portions, of course, can be bigger or smaller than the servings listed in the Food Guide Pyramid or on a food label" ("Food Portions," 1999). The portion was a quantity that illustrated how Americans controlled their food intake. Certain portions could be "better" or more "sensible" than others based on their comparison with the federally defined serving, as well as based on whether the eater has had "enough." The USDA's "How Much Are You Eating" (2002) publication urged Americans to "[r]esign from the 'clean your plate club'—when you've eaten enough, leave the rest" and "[p]ut sensible portions on your plate at the beginning of the meal, and don't take seconds."

The problem with the USDA's Food Guide Pyramid was that telling the public how many servings of each food group they ought to eat each day was not sufficient. The concept of a "serving" was confusing and unclear and gave the federal agencies cause for concern. If they were going to provide a layered quantitative framework for good eating, they needed to be clear as to exactly how much each quantity was. A USDA published *Nutrition Insights* newsletter writes:

Consumers appear to be confused about serving sizes—what they mean and how to use them. Complicating the problem are large portions of food that are becoming the norm in many eating establishments, which differ from the servings in the Food Guide Pyramid (FGP) and on the Nutrition Facts label on food packaging. For example, a large deli bagel might weigh 6 ounces (about 6 FGP servings of bread) while the ½ medium bagel on the Food Guide Pyramid weighs 1 ounce (about 1 serving of bread). With so much variation in portions of foods, it's easy for consumers to become confused about what serving sizes mean and how to use them ("Food Portions," 1999).

Every food choice, then, needed to fit a numeric portfolio: "portions" needed to become "servings" and "servings" needed to reflect the proper caloric category for the person. Educating the consumer could make the Food Guide Pyramid work as it should, and the USDA encouraged nutrition educators to "provide tips on how to visually estimate serving sizes," "explain how serving sizes differ from portion sizes," and "explain that Food Guide Pyramid servings are units of measure that are easy to use and understand" ("Food Portions," 1999). This mission for quantitative education illustrates the extent to which a discourse of quantification permeated every aspect of food and nutrition at the governmental level. At the USDA, every problem was quantified, as was every solution.

The popular press picked up on the USDA's criticism and call to action. They too, however, remained stuck in a quantitative rut and continued to define the problem in the terms set out by the USDA. Often, they reconceptualized the quantity of a serving into common physical items. Tara Parker-Pope of the *Wall Street Journal* writes:

> [O]ne of the biggest problems is that most people think a "serving" is how much they eat at one sitting. But a "serving" as defined by the government has nothing to do with how much a person should be served at any given time—it's simply a standard unit of measure, like a cup or a pint . . . a three ounce "serving" of meat, fish or poultry is about the size of a deck of cards. . . . Two tablespoons of peanut butter looks like a ping-pong ball. (Parker-Pope, 2003, p. D1)

Cooking Light magazine recommends a hand as the best gauge for determining the proper serving size. They provide sets of equivalents between servings of foods and various digits, fists, and palms. An ounce of cheese equals two fingers, a cupped hand equals a cup of dry cereal, and an open palm is a single serving of meat.[10]

These metaphors demonstrate the failure of a discourse of quantification to adequately describe how America ought to eat. While the USDA and the FDA relied on the calculated serving and portion to reduce ambiguity, metaphors like the palm and the ping-pong ball avail themselves to multiple interpretations and build on everyday lived experience. Government agencies took great pains in defining these quantities; demonstrating their inability to function outside of a language of scientific thought was all too easy. But the scientifically determined serving was quickly replaced by a metaphor. Simple linguistic tropes undermined the ability of a discourse of quantification to describe a complete epistemology of food by using more common modes of language that are better able to make sense of the human act of eating. Such metaphors also illustrated the importance and the necessity of human elements in discussions of food. Unfortunately, solving this problem of the serving and the portion meant increasing the importance of numbers in organizing America's relationship to food. Creating new quantities that co-opt words like "tradition" and "custom" denigrated the subjectivity of these terms and further abstracted the cultural aspects of food and eating.

Redefining Quality with Quantity: Walter Willett's Eating Right Pyramid

In the late 1990s Dr. Walter Willett, the chairman of the Department of Nutrition at the Harvard School of Public Health, also took issue with the USDA Pyramid. Willett's main grievance with the Food Pyramid was that it incorrectly designated "good" and "bad" foods, and that the designations were based on faulty science. Willett's (2001) criticisms culminate in his book *Eat, Drink, and Be Healthy,* in which he proposed replacing the USDA Pyramid with his own Eating Right Pyramid. Willett charges the USDA Food Guide Pyramid with being "wishy-washy, scientifically unfounded" and, at worst, the contributor to "overweight, poor health, and unnecessary early deaths" (p. 16). Willett complains that the USDA's 1992 guide is scientifically outdated, and was from its inception, and has disregarded advances in nutrition:

> For no-nonsense, rock-solid nutrition information, people often look to the Food Guide Pyramid. . . . [T]hat's a shame, because the USDA Pyramid is wrong. It was built on shaky scientific ground back in 1992. Since then it has been steadily eroded by new research from all parts of the globe. [But] the USDA Pyramid hasn't really changed in spite of important advances in what we know about nutrition and health. (pp. 15–16)

Willett's critique encompasses more than just general complaints about bad science. He points to several "holes in the USDA Pyramid" that were based on inadequate and incomplete scientific data (p. 18). As a result of these scientific holes, the Food Guide Pyramid incorrectly classifies the qualities of carbohydrates and fats. The Pyramid has an unwavering message: all starches are "good" and all fats are "bad." While the Pyramid's criteria for determining "good" and "bad" were entirely quantitative, it was not quantification that bothered Willett. Instead, he argues that the qualitative "good" and "bad" labels for carbohydrates and fats needed to be reclassified to reflect current scientific data. Willett's description of the problem, and his proposal for a solution, demonstrates that he too had fallen into the discursive trap of quantification.

One of Willett's major complaints about the USDA Pyramid is its treatment of fat. The Pyramid has an unequivocal message about fat: fat is bad. Fat and oils occupy the illicit acme of the Pyramid along with sweets.[11] But while sugar receives little attention in the USDA publication (it is after all, fat-free), fat gets plenty of press:

> The Pyramid focuses on fat because most Americans' diets are too high in fat. Following the Pyramid will help you keep your intake of total fat and saturated fat low. A diet low in fat will reduce your chances of getting certain diseases and help you maintain a healthy weight. ("Pyramid," 1992, preface)

The USDA guide recommends that Americans limit their daily fat intake to 30% of their calories, and do a "fat checkup" once in awhile to "keep you on the right track. If you find you are eating too much fat, choose lower fat foods more often" ("Pyramid," 1992, p. 12). The Pyramid publication suggests that the reduction of fat in the diet is one of "the best and simplest ways to lose weight" (p. 10). The USDA guide gives a brief description of the three kinds of fats found in foods: saturated, monounsaturated, and polyunsaturated. The guide recommends limiting saturated fats to 10% of daily calories, or one-third of the total fat intake, owing to saturated fats' connection with elevated cholesterol levels. Aside from a one-line nod to the perils of saturated fat, the guide makes no other distinction between the quality of certain fats or their sources.

Both the FDA and the USDA crafted the "All Fats Are Bad" message based on a rudimentary equation. Fats, as determined by Wilbur Atwater in the 19th century, are the most concentrated form of calories. One government publication entitled "Ways to Win at Weight Loss" reads: "Because fat is the most concentrated source of calories (9 calories per gram compared to 4 calories per gram for carbohydrate and protein), it is usually the focus of weight-management . . . limiting fat intake will likely limit calories as well" (Larkin, 1999). And so, the logic goes, since America *is* fat, it must be because Americans *eat* fat. Thus the USDA Pyramid imposes a numeric limit on fat to curb its insidious influence on America—a "good" diet consists of no more than 30% of "bad" fat.[12]

Because the USDA Food Pyramid's focus is on fat reduction in the American diet, starches, breads, and cereals—virtually fat-free in their basic forms—are the Pyramid's quantitative champions. The USDA represents the virtues of the bread, cereal, rice, and pasta group in the proportionally large base of the pyramid. According to the USDA, foods in the starch group are "an important source of energy, especially in low-fat diets" ("Pyramid," 1992, p. 19). For Americans keeping a tally of the foods they eat, this group represents the greatest number of servings per day: "At the base of the Food Guide Pyramid are breads, cereals, rice and pasta—all foods from grains. You need the most servings of these foods each day" (p. 5). The USDA establishes a quantitative rationale for the message that fat is "bad," and because the starchy base has relatively little fat, the USDA concurrently establishes the starch category's "goodness." The pyramid base is most "important," "providing vitamins, minerals and fiber" and this dispels the notion that starchy foods are fattening: "It's what you add to these foods or cook with them that adds most of the calories. For example: margarine or butter on bread, cream or cheese sauces on pasta, and the sugar and fat used with the flour in making cookies" (p. 19).[13] The pyramid base is "good" provided that the "bad" fats don't sully the celebrated fatlessness of the starch. The Food Guide Pyramid provides a chart of the number of grams of fat for several of the starch group items and encourages the consumption of breads, rolls, bagels, English muffins, rice, and pasta, all of which receive a special symbol to remind the eater that these are the best food choices. Defining the "quality" of the starchy base of the pyramid depends on the concurrent definition of the apex of fat.

One of Willett's main criticisms is that despite the USDA Pyramid's attempt to vilify *all* fats, they are not *all* worthy of vilification. Thus while all fats' caloric profile is 9 calories per gram, certain fats contain other nutrients, or have biological functions that make them "good":

> Few public health messages are as powerful and as persistent as this one: Fat is bad. Over the past four decades, fat has become a kind of dietary Public Enemy Number One, a food feared for its ability to cause disease and even kill. . . . In spite of the scorn heaped upon dietary fat . . . *some fats are good for you, and it is important to include these good fats in your diet.* (Willett, 2001, p. 56, emphasis in original)

In *Eat, Drink, and Be Healthy*, Willett sets out to redefine notions of good and bad with respect to fats. He begins with debunking the "intuitive" notion perpetuated by the USDA that eating more fat makes you fatter. Willett points out that over the last 20 years Americans have reduced their fat intake from 40% to 34% but the average weight of Americans and the percentage of the population that are overweight and obese has increased in that same time. Willett also dispels the myth that high fat intake is an indicator of high levels of heart disease, and points to the Seven Countries Study, which indicated that Cretans who had the highest intake of fat (almost all of it from olive oil) had the lowest incidence of heart disease among the various countries.

But to redefine the qualitative concepts of good and bad fat Willett heads to the laboratory, in efforts to teach the reader the chemical composition, the carbon geometry, and the stereoisomeric differences between saturated and unsaturated fats. By learning more about the science of fats, Willett develops a set of criteria by which judgments of good and bad are made possible. Willett-defined-good fats are mono- and polyunsaturated fats. These fats are worthy of the "good" classification for a variety of reasons, and Willet includes scientific data and lists of numbers and graphs to validate his claims. Monounsaturated fats (of which sources include olive oil, canola oil, peanut oil, avocados, and most nuts) raise levels of high-density lipoproteins (HDL), the good cholesterol, and simultaneously lower levels of low-density lipoproteins (LDL), the bad cholesterol:

> LDL is often referred to as the bad cholesterol. When your bloodstream picks up too many of these particles, they can end up in the wrong places, especially inside cells that line the blood vessels. . . . In contrast, HDL particles sponge up excess cholesterol from the lining of blood vessels and elsewhere and carry it off to the liver for disposal. . . . The best cholesterol profile is one with a low level of LDL cholesterol and a high level of HDL. Good fats can improve the cholesterol profile. (Willett, 2001, pp. 66–69)

Good fats for Willett are ones that have a well-defined scientific and quantitatively assessed function. Good fats can make measured improvements in health, and these improvements can be identified, charted, and objectively assessed. There is one class of polyunsaturated fats that Willett calls special. He claims that these n-3 (or Omega-3) fatty acids deserve individual attention because they carry with them a panoply of health benefits. Readers are encouraged to select foods with high levels of these n-3 fatty acids, and Willett provides them with an itemized list of foods ranked in order of their concentration of these fats. According to Willett, making fat the absolute "bad" nutritional component because of the simple association with its quantitative caloric concentration is wrong, misleading, and dangerous to American public health. Willett's solution to this problem, however, is to rely on quantification to provide the eater with more numbers upon which they should based their qualitative judgments.

According to Willett, fats are not the only misclassified foods in the Food Guide Pyramid. Another of his criticisms strikes at the very base of the pyramid: the "good" and low-fat foundation of starch. Just as he had done with the unequivocal "fat is bad" message, Willett also takes aim at "all carbohydrates are good." In *Eat, Drink, and Be Healthy*, not all carbohydrates are created equal. Willet is quick to point out that the good starch designation is simplistic, and he fears that such a designation created the overconsumption of all carbohydrates—regardless of their quality:

> The [other] big problem is that little attention has been paid to the *types* of carbohydrates we eat. A diet high in refined carbohydrates that are quickly digested and absorbed can have damaging consequences. These include higher levels of blood sugar, insulin, and triglycerides, and lower levels of HDL cholesterol. In other words, more cardiovascular disease and diabetes. But these kinds of carbohydrates are strongly promoted by the USDA Food Guide Pyramid. (p. 86)

Just as with fats, Willett uses a discourse of quantification and the authority of science to define the notion of "quality" carbohydrates, and introduces a new assessment tool for measuring the goodness in each type of carbohydrate. Good carbohydrates are complex carbohydrates with a low glycemic index. The glycemic index is a measurement of the speed with which carbohydrates enter the bloodstream. Low glycemic indices (GIs) mean that foods will release their component sugars more slowly into the bloodstream thereby preventing spikes in insulin and keeping hunger at bay for longer periods of time. By using the glycemic index as a quantitative rhetorical tool, Willett argues that good foods are those that have GIs less than 100, a numeric standard that functions in the same way as the Recommended Daily Allowances established by the USDA in the 1940s. Above a certain GI, foods are bad, and below a certain GI, foods are good. These good carbohydrates "protect against diabetes," "cut the chances of heart disease by about one-third," "improve [gastrointestinal] health," and "may keep cancer at bay" (pp. 96–97). Willett buttresses this justification for eating good carbohydrates with data and studies from the *Journal of the American Medical Association*, and the *American Journal of Clinical Nutrition* and represents the GIs of good carbohydrates using graphs, charts, and diagrams. In providing this sort of evidence Willett uses the same topos of quantity in his attempts to encourage change.

Scientific oversights on the part of the USDA created an ideal space for Willett to critique the absolutist notions of good and bad. The possibility existed to trouble the quantitative understanding of qualitative terms and to propose an alternative approach to using numbers to judge the quality of a food. Instead, Willett's criticism of the USDA Pyramid mimicked, reproduced, and tweaked its quantitative discourse. He relied on the established topos of quantity, the USDA's scientific validation for their model of how to eat and even their iconographic conduit, the pyramid. Thus, in response to the USDA's "shaky" pyramid, Willett proposes his *own* pyramid, the Healthy Eating Pyramid to counter the federal government's "scientifically unfounded" nutrition advice. He pronounces his diet "based on the best scientific evidence" that "fixes the fundamental flaws of the USDA Pyramid and helps you make better choices about what to eat" (pp. 16–17).

Willett's Healthy Eating Pyramid reflects his effort to change the perception of certain fats from bad to good and certain carbohydrates from good to bad. The base of his pyramid consists of whole grain foods and "plants oils, including olive, canola, soy, corn, sunflower, peanut, and other vegetable oils" (p. 7). Willett insists that his pyramid "isn't a single cute idea dolled up in a catchy graphic." Instead "it is the distillation of evidence from many different lines of research" (p. 17). He is quick to dismiss the "catchy graphic," but uses its designed quantitative function of proportionality to relay his own message about nutrition. The USDA had crafted the message that the base of the pyramid, its largest visible proportion, houses the "good" foods, the foods that Americans ought to consume most frequently, and are the best for them. Willett, by including certain (scientifically validated) fats in the base of his own pyramid, relied on the same visual and spatial argument for "quality."

In addition to using the quantitative message of the spatialization of the pyramid, Willett relies on a discourse of quantification to get his own message of quality across to the public. According to Willett, part of the problem of the current nutritional messages is the ill-defined concept of quality. Therefore, his criticisms of the USDA Food Pyramid, however scientifically valid they may be, demonstrate his own incarceration in a quantitative discourse, and in the topos of quantity that the USDA ascribed to food a hundred years earlier. On the surface, the message of Willett's food guide looks different from the USDA's. Willett's Healthy Eating Pyramid debunks several of the USDA's fundamental messages, but rhetorically the message is no different.

Quantifying Lifestyle: Red Wine, Heart Disease, and the Mediterranean Diet

One of the USDA's goals in the Food Guide Pyramid is the reduction of heart disease. Included as part of the guide are the *Dietary Guidelines for Americans*, which the U.S. Department of Agriculture and the Department of Health and Human Services publish jointly. The guidelines are the basis of federal nutrition policy and inform the messages of the Food Guide Pyramid. These guidelines encourage diet modification for the express purpose of the reduction of heart disease. The Pyramid correlates heart disease with consumption of fat and cholesterol, and recommends that eaters curb their intake of foods that contain these components in order to reduce their risk.

> Dietary cholesterol, as well as saturated fat, raises blood cholesterol levels in many people, increasing their risk for heart disease. Some health authorities recommend that dietary cholesterol be limited to an average of 300 mg or less per day. To keep dietary cholesterol to this level, follow the Food Guide Pyramid, keeping your total fat to the amount that's right for you. ("Pyramid," 1992, p. 15)

Constructing fat as the problem was not new for the USDA—they had already made fat culpable for America's expanding waistline. By placing a numeric limit on fat, and cholesterol, the USDA hoped to reduce the incidence of heart disease.

Around the time of the release of the Food Guide Pyramid, new information about coronary heart disease and diet challenged the USDA's no fat–no heart disease correlation. In 1992, the British medical journal *The Lancet* published "Wine, Alcohol, Platelets, and the French Paradox for Coronary Heart Disease." The article's abstract stated that "the mortality from coronary heart disease is much lower in France than it is in other industrialized countries, even though the French eat as much fat as individuals in other countries. The consumption of wine by the French could explain their low death rates from heart disease" (Renaud and de Lorgeril, 1992, p. 1523). Despite greater fat, saturated fat, and cholesterol consumption, the French seemed to be able to enjoy their triple-cream brie and remain heart healthy, provided they washed their meals down with red wine. The study chided America's rigid approach to fat consumption and their correlation of high fat consumption with heart disease:

> Dietary habits consistent with protection from CHD (coronary heart disease) have been considered too restrictive . . . however,

the diet in Toulouse, France, is varied and characterized by low consumption of butter and high consumption of bread, vegetables, fruits, cheese, vegetable fat and wine—i.e., a Mediterranean-type diet. (p. 1523)[14]

On American soil, it was the viniferous component of this French Paradox that was most intriguing to the press and caused the most controversy. The *Lancet* study provided incentive for some to challenge the USDA's dietary advice. Could red wine be what America needed to reduce coronary heart disease? For a country with a history of prohibition, encouraging the consumption of alcohol was a difficult thing to do regardless of the reported health benefits.

After the release of the study that pointed to the healthfulness of the Mediterranean Diet, wine became a hot topic in the press and a political problem for the American government. It was only a few years earlier, in 1989, that Congress passed a law requiring wine labels to print alcohol consumption warnings. In spite of the evidence for the health benefits of moderate alcohol consumption, the USDA and the American press could not bring themselves to advocate the consumption of wine. The USDA Food Guide Pyramid encouraged moderation when drinking alcoholic beverages because they were "the cause of many health problems and accidents and can lead to addiction" ("Pyramid," 1992, p. 1).

In the years that followed the *Lancet* study two types of responses emerged from the press. The first focused on the mystery of the French Paradox and perpetuated gastronomic stereotypes of the French. Articles constructed the French culture as indulgent and irresponsible. The French smoked too much and ate meals of foie gras. Americans often attributed their low heart disease to luck and repeatedly highlighted the mystery of the paradox:

How can those French get away with eating triple-cream brie and *sauce béarnaise* and still have one of the lowest rates of heart disease in the industrialized world? (Reynolds, 1993, p. 46)

When international surveys in the 1980s showed substantially lower rates of coronary heart disease in France than in other industrialized nations, scientists were puzzled. How could this be true in the land of pâté de foie gras and Gauloises, burgundy and béarnaise sauce? This contradiction is called the French Paradox. (Thomas, 1994, pp. 4–5)

Americans have been muddling over the merits of merlot and chablis ever since 1991, when the *New York Times* and *60 Minutes* carried stories on the so-called French paradox—the ability of the French to eat gobs of buttery sauces and foie gras while avoiding heart disease. (Brownlee and Barnett, 1994, p. 62)

According to the press, it was bad enough that the French had delicious creamy cakes, they could eat them too, providing they drank red wine. As *USA Today* pointed out, "people in France eat more rich, fatty foods than those in the U.S. The French exercise less and smoke more than Americans. Yet the so-called French Paradox is that the death rate from heart disease is markedly lower in France than in other industrialized countries, including America. It just doesn't seem fair" (Hackman, 1998, pp. 58–60).

While some were concerned with the ideological construction of French culture, others began to quantify one of the more "cultural" aspects of the French Paradox, red wine. Solving the paradox meant eliminating uncertainty and creating more data, using scientific terms and a discourse of quantification. If science could determine *why* red wine had such a magical effect on the heart and arteries, then science could determine exactly *how much* red wine we needed to drink to be healthy. Chemists and doctors were called upon to isolate the compounds in wine that were the agents of good health. Thus, instead of focusing on *how, where*, and *why* people drank, science focused on *who was drinking, how much they drank*, and *what was in what they were drinking*. Rhetorically, the quantification of wine reduced it to chemical compounds and relied on the persuasive topos of quantity to persuade the USDA of wine's beneficial aspects. Instead of treating wine as a gastronomic entity whose consumption could enhance our eating experience, as well as our health, science abducted wine from the subjective experience of drinking. Wine became the subject of intense scientific scrutiny, analyzed in the lab to determine what it contained that made the French so healthy.

One group of researchers singled out trans-resveratrol (Res) as the explanation for the Mediterranean Diet's cardio-protective effects and as containing anticancer properties:

We showed that Res was a potent inhibitor of both NF-kB activation and NF-kB-dependent gene expression . . . our results suggest that the major mechanism whereby Res blocks NF-kB activity is through the inhibition of IKK activity. This finding may partly explain how Res could inhibit oncogenic and inflammatory diseases in human beings. (Holmes-McNary et al. 2000, p. 3477)

Another study isolated phenolic antioxidants that "reduced plate-let aggregation" when subjects consumed 200 milliliters of red wine (Seigneur et al., 1990; Waterhouse, 1994). Scientists analyzed phenols even further and reduced them to active biochemical agents called flavinoids. One study tested red wines to determine which grape varietals had the greatest concentration of flavinoids: cabernet sauvignon, petite syrah, and pinot noir were deemed the best, and merlots, red zinfandels, and white wines, which have the lowest concentration of flavinoids, were the least beneficial. A discourse of quantification allowed the public to judge the quality of a wine not on its bouquet, its region, or its vintage, but on its concentration of flavinoids. Although the word "flavinoid" does not share an etymological origin with "flavor," it is difficult not to consider "flavinoid" as a scientized stand-in for "flavor"—a signifier that strips "flavor" of its subjective flair, replacing it with a discrete and countable quantity. Finding the "right" wine no longer meant pairing it with the right food for a superlative taste experience. Instead, a "good" bottle of wine had sufficient flavinoids with proven health benefits. While the French were enjoying the quality of the experience of drinking wine, they were oblivious to wine's *actual* benefits:

> A fine bottle of French wine is renowned around the word for contributing to the pleasure of a good meal and company. The real value to the French, though, may be due to certain heart-healthy substances in the wine they consume, particularly red wine. Scientists now believe that natural chemical compounds in red wine called biologically active flavinoids may confer important health benefits to the heart and blood vessels, and help explain the French Paradox. (Hackman, 1998, p. 58)

Frequently, consumers were called upon to substitute red wine with grape juice or raisins. One company even went as far as extracting flavinoids and creating a tablet called the CardioFlav 500, for "those who cannot consume alcohol" ("French Paradox," 2000). Instead of drinking wine, America could pop a pill, with the same flavorful "bite" as red wine. Science gave America a quantified reason for drinking wine, and then eliminated the need to drink it all together.

These two strategies for dealing with the French Paradox illustrate an odd alignment of science and ethics around questions of food consumption. The first strategy clearly assumes a kind of decadence, hedonism, and self-indulgence among the French, and these characteristics are the grounds for a critique of their lifestyle. The French lack restraint and they practice indulgence—this is their moral failing. The paradox arises because they are not punished for that failing and instead seem to thrive. The second strategy, of scientifically accounting for French health, assumes a position of ethical neutrality, and objectivity—as all science seems to do. But still the French are made to seem inadequate because they do not know the real reason for their health. The pose of neutrality is designed to elevate American explanations for drinking above French "cultural" explanations. These scientific accounts have the authority of a different kind of evidence and justification and, therefore, they escape the possibility of association with hedonism and decadence that can often accompany drinking. By switching from a subjective language of taste in describing wine (a language that could not possibly account for health benefits) to a scientized and quantified language, the press is able to escape questions about the ethics of drinking while maintaining the guise of American superiority.

With the French Paradox study in the *Lancet* articulating the "Mediterranean-type diet," an organization concerned with American nutrition and food called the Oldways Preservation and Exchange Trust began working on creating official Mediterranean Diet guidelines. Oldways evolved from the American Institute of Wine and Food founded by Julia Child and Robert Mondavi in 1981. The trust was committed to "promoting healthy eating, traditional foodways, and sustainable food choices with effective, common-sense education programs" (Oldways, 2001). In the summer of 1994, delegates from the Oldways Preservation and Exchange Trust, the Harvard School of Public Health, and the World Health Organization attended a conference called Wine's Place at a Healthy Table. At the conference, Oldways released their own Mediterranean Diet guidelines: "a panel of authorities . . . will unveil its new guidelines for a healthy diet, based on Mediterranean cultures. It features lots of pasta, couscous, bulgur, yoghurt, olive oil—and one or two glasses of wine a day" (Miller, 1994, p. B1).

The Oldways Trust called the Mediterranean Diet a "proven cultural model for healthy eating" and contrasted it with the "theoretical construct" of the USDA's Pyramid:

[T]he USDA pyramid was constructed against the backdrop of a national dietary pattern which is known to contribute to heart disease, cancer, and other chronic disease which persist at high rates in this country. Without the existence of a "home-grown" time-tested cultural model of healthy eating on which to base the USDA Pyramid, this graphic is by definition a more speculative document. (Oldways, 2001)

Oldways' Mediterranean Diet attempts to introduce a new topos to encourage people to eat in a particular way: culture. Those who adhered to the Mediterranean Diet would be following a "home-grown" tradition that had the semantic weight of years of heart-healthy Mediterranean people. But they too were trapped in a discourse of quantification.

It appeared that the topos of culture might provide a different discourse with which to discuss food—a discourse that discussed *how* Mediterraneans ate instead of *what* they ate. The very concept of a healthy diet belonging to a region and a culture begged questions of lifestyle, seasonality, and qualitative aspects of eating. But while Oldways' Mediterranean Diet may have created the opportunity for a discursive space in which one could articulate food and eating using an alternative qualitative discourse, the fascination with the science behind red wine reduced the diet to its objective and quantitative features:

> In the Mediterranean tradition, wine was enjoyed in moderation and normally with meals and typically within a family context. For men, moderation is defined as one to two glasses of wine per day. Moderate alcohol consumption for men appears not only to lower the risk of heart disease but also to reduce overall mortality. (Oldways, 1994, p. 6)

Here, Oldways talks about tradition, family, and the idiosyncratic concepts of moderation. In the Mediterranean, it is not necessary to define and delineate these concepts. However, in their dietary advice to their American counterparts, they *quantify* moderation. For "men," they invent a numeric baseline for what constitutes moderation—one to two glasses of wine per day. While in Europe, wine may have been part of the cultural experience of eating, in American discourse, wine and its benefits were something to be abstracted and counted. Importing a gastronomic lifestyle because it was healthier meant that the culture had to somehow demonstrate, in a quantifiable way, why it was healthier. Attempts to use the topos of culture to encourage Americans to eat in a particular way only resulted in the redefinition of that topos using a discourse of quantification. Mediterranean cultures and the pleasures of a glass of wine had little to do with flavinoids, phenols, and trans-resveratrol. But in order to make sense of a lifestyle that was incommensurable with American discourses of food and eating, the qualitative aspects of culture had to be quantified. Mediterranean populations may have other sources of knowledge that construct and inform their daily diet like history, tradition, and culture. But the reliability of this knowledge was suspect until it was validated by science and redefined using a discourse of quantification.

The taboo and complex subject of alcohol consumption in America forced the media to reduce wine to a chemical compound. In so doing, they completely missed some of the fundamental features of the *act of consumption* itself that explained the paradox. A scant number of articles mentioned the physical activity levels of the French subjects of the *Lancet* study (they were farmers and thus had an active lifestyle). Few mentioned the French tradition of longer relaxed meals or the timing of their intake (larger meals were generally taken midday and often lasted two or more hours). Almost none of the articles mentioned that the original *Lancet* study stated that although the French eat foie gras and "gourmet foods," it was on special occasions, and their diet remained heterogeneous and "characterized by low consumption of butter and high consumption of bread, vegetables, fruit, cheese, vegetable fat and wine" (Renaud and de Lorgeril, 1992, p. 1524). Instead, the American media took to creating caricatures of the French. But the French ate a wider variety of foods, exercised more, and ate their meals slowly, often enjoying a glass or two of wine. This was not a paradox; it was simply a way of life that was incommensurable with the American habits of consumption. Very few articles mentioned the social factors that correlate to moderate alcohol intake—class, culture, and education—that also affect dietary intake and coronary risk. Oddly enough, lower levels of stress that result from a glass of wine were never mentioned as a possibility of reduced heart disease either. Only one researcher, Dr. Curtis Ellison, mentioned that "it may not be the amount of wine that they drink but the pattern in which they consume it, in moderation and with meals" (Thomas, 1994, p. 5). There was thus little critical examination of *how* the French eat, how the act of consumption is actually performed. According to the press, an American could not imagine spending two or three hours eating a larger meal at lunch, having a few glasses of wine and a dose of relaxed conversation or a stroll after their meal.

In this context, science is being used to demarcate a threshold within which an activity is acceptable. This kind of demarcation requires a clearly specifiable quantity, an abstraction not tied in any way to culture or tradition or people. Such a quantity allows for comparison between and across different populations. The studies that try to draw this line must, however, suggest that by staying on one side of the line the drinker receives considerable health benefits, while crossing that line leads to serious health risks. For example, a 2000 article from the *Annals of Internal Medicine* suggests that "compared with no alcohol, up to 21 drinks per

week" significantly reduced the risk of coronary disease, while consumption of more than 21 drinks per week increases one's risk of death from
cancer. The line between reducing risk of heart disease and increasing
risk of cancer leaves little margin for error. In such a case, alcohol is
either beneficial or harmful; it is never neutral (Grønbæk et al., 2000. p.
411). Heart disease and cancer are just two among many ailments that
wine consumption could affect positively or negatively. In 2005 the *New
England Journal of Medicine* reported that moderate red wine consumption
in women, here defined as 15.0 grams of alcohol per day or one drink,
resulted in better cognitive function than that of nondrinkers or drinkers
who drank in excess of moderation, and that as the patients aged, the
moderate drinkers were more likely to retain cognitive function than others
(Stampfer et al., 2005, p. 245). In this instance, consumption of alcohol
had its benefits, providing the patient consumed it in the prescribed or
dosed manner. Wine consumption among men is treated in the same way
in the journal *Diabetes*. Men who consumed 15–29 grams of alcohol per
day (an amount the journal considers "moderate") were less likely to be
affected by type 2 diabetes (36% less likely) than those who consumed no
alcohol (Conigrave et al., 2001, p. 2390). In this case it was the routine
of drinking wine that offered the health benefits. Drinkers who consumed
moderate amounts daily reaped the greatest benefits. In fact, the greater
the number of days of the week the patients drank the prescribed amount
(not more or less), the lower their risk of type 2 diabetes. In this case it
wasn't just the amount of wine that created the demarcation, it was also
the method of drinking the prescribed amount that created "health."

To return to the outcome of the 1994 conference Wine's Place at
a Healthy Table, the Mediterranean Diet guidelines were released as a
European counterpart to the USDA's Food Pyramid. But the Mediterranean Diet resembled the Food Guide Pyramid in shape only. It had not
quantified the portions per day of the various food groups that must be
taken to ensure health. The diet merely encouraged daily consumption of
fruits, vegetables, legumes, nuts, starches, olive oil, cheese, yogurt, exercise,
and wine (Miller, 1994, p. B1). Advocates of the diet faced some harsh
criticism, mostly from centers on addiction and substance abuse, as well
as the United States National Institute on Alcohol Abuse and Alcoholism.
The Mediterranean Diet defenders took pains to point out that it was
"moderate" consumption of wine that reaped the most health benefits, and
that wine was just one factor that added to overall good health—hence
the need to determine the line between the quantity that was beneficial
and the quantity that was harmful. Dr. Andrew Ball of the WHO stated
his surprise at the WHO's involvement in the Mediterranean Diet, and
pointed out that "moderate" wine consumption was a cultural tradition

in Europe, but that that sensibility and control may not exist in other cultures (Miller, 1994, p. B1).

The storied history of alcohol consumption in America had left it to be governed along with other lethal entities in the Federal Bureau of Alcohol, Tobacco, and Firearms (BATF). Alcohol consumption was stigmatizing, not salubrious; drinkers were destined to become drunks, not cultured or healthy. Perhaps American history would be the biggest roadblock in accepting alcohol as part of a healthy daily routine. However, in 1995, with scientific and epidemiological evidence mounting, the American government made a huge policy change toward alcohol consumption. The updated version of the USDA-published *Dietary Guidelines for Americans* stated that "current evidence suggests that moderate drinking is associated with a lower risk for coronary heart disease in some individuals" (USDA, 1995). Despite the long list of "risk groups" who were to ignore the dietary advice including people less than 21 years of age, family members with a history of alcoholism, and women who were trying to conceive, this declaration was a boon for the status of alcohol in America. It was only a few years prior that the USDA had stated that alcohol had "no net health benefit" and was "not recommended" as part of a healthy American diet (USDA, 1992). What made the American government modify its position on alcohol is unknown, but they could not ignore the national and international scientific evidence in favor of moderate alcohol consumption any longer. Despite the fact that the statement was made about alcohol in general, the press chose wine as the exemplar. In January 1996, an article about red wine consumption in the magazine *Newsweek* asked, with its title, "To Your Health?" and showed a large glass of red wine as the accompanying picture. In the eyes of the popular press, wine was not only the magic bullet, but it was the magic bullet that directly and rationally challenged American prohibitionist history. The press still preferred to downplay the importance of the lifestyle aspects that accompanied red wine consumption among the French: exercise, stress-free meals, and longer, more attentive dining.

Magazines like *Forbes*, *Better Nutrition*, *Prevention*, and *American Fitness* all reported on the health benefits of wine heralding its polyphenols, salicylic acid, and flavonoids as panaceas conquering cancer, heart disease, and age-related macular degeneration as well as lowering overall mortality. For example, *Forbes* magazine writes that wine can reduce the risk of cancer and heart disease stating that "the protection probably comes from chemicals in the wine called polyphenols, compounds that have been shown to fight cancer as well as heart disease" (1997, p. 90). *Better Nutrition* cited a study that found that "a glass of wine every once in a while actually protects health, specifically vision, in the long run" and that those who engaged in the "moderate use of wine" had the lowest incidences of age-related macular degeneration (Dolby, 1998, p. 16). Few articles mentioned the aspect of dietary variety and routine exercise in the lives of the French and most still marveled at red wine's apparent "canceling out" of the deleterious effects of indulging in foie gras. Ideologically, the French continued to "lead unhealthy lives, filled with fatty foods and excessive smoking" (Hackman, 1998, p. 58). The *Lancet* study provided incentive for some to challenge the USDA's dietary advice. Could red wine be what America needed to reduce coronary heart disease, cancer, and vision problems? For a country with a history of prohibition, encouraging the consumption of alcohol was difficult to do regardless of the reported health benefits.

Domestic winemakers used the mounting scientific evidence to lobby the government for the ability to print health claims on wine labels. In 1996, the Wine Institute of America proposed the following statement to the BATF to be printed on wine bottle labels: "The proud people who made this wine encourage you to consult your family doctor about the health effects of moderate wine consumption" (BATF, 1999). The BATF took issue with the word "moderate" because they thought it sounded like a reason to drink. Known teetotaler Strom Thurmond, a Republican from South Carolina, appealed to then treasury secretary Robert Rubin to reject the Wine Institute's request outright. But because of the mounting scientific evidence for moderate alcohol consumption to decrease heart disease, Thurmond was ignored. On February 5, 1999, a BATF press release announced that they had approved labels with modified versions of the Wine Institute's proposals. On October 25, 1999, the BATF invited comments on the policy approving the health statements. Due to a lack of response, they announced on December 9, 1999, that they would hold public hearings on the issue of health claims on labels of wine. These hearings were subsequently cancelled, and by January 2000 the BATF had shelved the proposal. It was only a few years earlier, in 1989, that Congress passed a law requiring wine labels to print alcohol consumption warnings. In spite of the evidence for the health benefits of moderate alcohol consumption, the American federal government could not bring itself to advocate the consumption of wine. The USDA Food Guide Pyramid continued to encourage "moderation" when drinking alcoholic beverages because they were "the cause of many health problems and accidents and can lead to addiction" ("Pyramid," 1996, p. 1).

This story illustrates several key features of the relationship between science and the public regarding food and drink. First, the controversy over the meaning of moderation indicates that science controls the process of definition. Furthermore, the definition of moderation can only be rendered in quantitative terms so that it can be applied to as many people in as many circumstances as possible, while avoiding subjective cultural renderings of what "moderate" may mean. Second, this definition of moderation stands as a new ethical mandate able to prescribe courses of action while remaining insulated from cultural criticism. Third, such a definition also serves to create two kinds of populations—those that drink in a healthy fashion and those that drink in an unhealthy fashion. Both categories of people can be understood as patients. The first category is engaged in the task of warding off the inevitable development of disease through good choices. The second category develops diseases and illnesses because of behaviors like excessive drinking. Both categories are responsible for their own health and responsible for monitoring the line between behavior that is beneficial and behavior that is harmful. Members of the first category are good patients working in tandem with public health officials, while members of the second category are irresponsible. This division certifies an understanding of health as prevention.

Walter Willett also deals with the difficulty of determining the meaning of "moderate" in *Eat, Drink, and Be Healthy*. Willett shies away from endorsing any level of alcohol consumption, and claims that the health benefits experienced by those that live in the Mediterranean are a result of other factors beyond wine (2001, pp. 136–137). But, if one must drink wine, one must drink it in moderation. To determine the exact numerical equivalent of moderation, one must perform a risk-benefit calculation. Depending on the person, this calculation could produce different results, based on family history of high cholesterol or alcoholism, weight, age, and so forth. In any case, the health benefits of moderate drinking can easily be achieved from other things, like exercise. As one of the leading authorities on public health, Willett's recommendation to perform a risk-benefit calculation, as the only reasonable way to draw the line between healthy consumption and unhealthy consumption, is a recommendation to act more like a scientist. In other words, to "eat, drink, and be healthy" is to learn how to use a discourse of quantification to determine what and how much to drink and eat.

From such a perspective, a "healthy" drinker is one who adheres to the latest scientific evidence regarding the role of flavonoids in preventing heart disease or regarding the risk of alcohol in developing cancer. Being "healthy" becomes a particular kind of enumerated judgment—it refers to the capacity to make risk-benefit calculations, "how much" becomes a stand-in for "how good." The construction of a healthy drinker in response to the French Paradox creates another mechanism to make moral evaluations of those who drink too much. In this case, the moral failure is a failure to be adequately scientific and mathematical. But this notion of the scientific and mathematical drinker is part of a larger tradition of practicing restraint, self-control, and self-discipline. The scientized justification for such a position is the latest in a long line of recommendations for this sort of behavior that date back to the origins of Stoic philosophy and Christian virtue. In the public understanding of the benefits of drinking wine, science teaches ethics and prescribes codes of conduct, and it is an ethics of restraint, self-control, and self-discipline—the same ethics that underpin the life in the laboratory that produces the justifications for wine's health benefits.

The scientization of wine, therefore, employs a rhetoric of demarcation in order to prescribe correct drinking habits. The 2005 *Dietary Guidelines for Americans* published by the USDA states "those who choose to drink alcoholic beverages should do so *sensibly* and in *moderation*" (p. 44, emphasis mine). Such a move associates the public role of science with a long tradition of ethical imperatives. In this case, as a normalizing tactic, science shares a great deal with both the Stoic and the Christian traditions (Peters, 2005). Ultimately, the science behind wine teaches a kind of rationalized prohibition. Instead of prohibiting drinking, one attempts to regulate the quantity of drink consumed.

Three Critiques, One Mode of Communication

The American response to the French Paradox is, in part, a story of the development and extension of scientized and numeric language as applied to food. It is not the numbers themselves, nor the molecular descriptions, that are new, but it is their application to an object of consumption almost always described in moral, cultural, traditional, or experiential terms that is new. There is a civic and ethical function to the development and use of such a scientific/quantitative language, a function that has long underpinned American conceptions of democratic life. As John Durham Peters puts it:

> As a set of communication practices, quantification specifically claims to establish open relations among colleagues, present clear standards of evaluation, and subject opinions to facts. It imagines a community of enlightened, altruistic people that bow before the best data. (2005, p. 196)

Peters claims that scientific practices go hand-in-hand with democracy because of their commitment to revision, openness, and impartiality. What is unique in this case, however, is that scientific practices of counting, and scientific talk in numbers and data, are mimicked in the recommendations for consumption of wine. In other words, we are encouraged to drink like scientists, by counting. Once one's understanding of wine has been scientized and enumerated, then one's behavior will likely mimic the behavior of scientists in the lab. This is the goal of public understanding of the science of wine.

If one drinks like a scientist, then one is insulated from ethical condemnation. The story of American responses to the French Paradox makes this clear. Moreover, the development and use of a quantitative and scientific language regarding wine allows for the invention of a group, or population, of "healthy drinkers." The members of this virtuous category are easily celebrated for their self-restraint and juxtaposed with alcoholics. Numbers create populations (Foucault, 1994; Hacking, 1990), and those populations are then provided with the tools to make ethical evaluations of their own conduct (Miller, 1993). What, on its surface, appears to be a move away from moral questions and toward health questions, is actually a move toward an ethics that celebrates the self-restraint of a scientist, now drinker, who knows the objective line between healthy and dangerous. In the example of the French Paradox, the discourse of quantification begins to do more and more qualitative work.

Examining alternatives to, and critiques of, the USDA Food Guide Pyramid demonstrates the extent to which a discourse of quantification permeated discussions of the American diet. No part of the eating process was spared from calculation, measurement, and science. The USDA and FDA confusion over serving and portion regulations hijacked the language of occasion, custom, and tradition, and forced it into tidy quantitative calculations. The fact that the critics of the Pyramid did not expect the USDA to address intractable problems around social and cultural traditions and customs illustrates the control that a discourse of quantification exercised over the American government's conceptions of eating. Walter Willett saw problems with the USDA Pyramid and identified qualitative terms that the USDA used incorrectly. However, instead of troubling the quantitative epistemology, Willett redefined it in his own terms. A discourse of quantification had permeated Willett's discussion of how to eat to such an extent that subjective terms like "good" and "bad" were defined by objective, scientific, and measured language. By redefining words and respatializing the USDA's quantitative Pyramid, Willett demonstrates that while he was critical of the USDA, he could not conceive of his critique with alternative discursive means. For Willett, the problem with the American diet was not the topos of quantity that buttressed the epistemology of quality. The problem was that said epistemology was doomed to fail, if it did not have accurate and timely science to shore it up.

The example of the French Paradox, the Mediterranean Diet, and the role of red wine in these Pyramid alternatives demonstrate how a discourse of quantification works to co-opt the qualitative and cultural component of a diet. Oldways Trust and the American press's treatment of red wine abstracts it from its context in order to calculate and theorize how and why it contributes to a healthier diet—that is, one where there is a lower incidence of heart disease. These critiques use the topos of culture to encourage America to drink wine—but they do not encourage America to enjoy it. Because wine was the suspected panacea, it was subject to scientific scrutiny and quantitative analysis. When the quantity of wine consumption in a healthy diet was determined to fall under the rubric of discretionary "in moderation," Oldways was quick to calculate and numerically define "moderation"—one to two glasses of wine per day. This final example of a discourse of quantification's appropriation of a dietary component with a cultural and geographic history demonstrates its deficiencies. Food policy and nutrition initiatives are unable to address subjective components like lifestyle unless they are treated numerically and scientifically. Thus, the role of red wine in Mediterranean culture, the history of this beverage in the region, and even oeno-gastronomic traditions of Western Europe are subjected to calculation. What is missing, however, is the description of these qualitative components, the incalculable aspects of how food and wine fit into the daily rhythms of life—how culture, history, and geography play a role in a good diet, and can help redefine notions of quality using alternative languages. In what follows, I address these languages, or discourses of taste, and how they employ alternative topoi and criteria for crafting an epistemology of quality.

Chapter Five

Talking about Taste

Alternatives to a Discourse of Quantification

In the past four chapters I have shown how a discourse of quantification—adopted by the USDA in the late 1800s—forms the basis for much persuasive communication about food. This quantitative discourse has become part of food, imparting constitutive qualities that are inexorably linked to a food itself. For the USDA, the makers of nutrition policy and food guidance in America, the emergence and development of a discourse of quantification meant that an apple was not simply an apple. An apple was 5 grams of fiber, 80 calories, or one serving of fruit. This discourse of quantification extended itself and became layered such that numbers came to refer to other numbers and numeric standards. Judging food became dependent upon quantities and how they compared to standards. The apple's 5 grams of fiber made it a good source when compared to the USDA dietary fiber charts. In this case, the qualitative judgment of "good" came from having more fiber. As I have shown, "more" does not always mean "good." As food continued to be the subject of scientific analysis, and physiology labs continued to analyze people, the discovery was that in some cases "more" was "bad." For example, scientists determined that a high intake of saturated fat was one possible cause of heart disease—more fat equated to more heart disease, thus fat became bad, and less of it became good.

If one were to refer to the quantitative messages of the USDA Food Guide Pyramid, a thick, marbled, juicy Delmonico steak with a port wine glaze, hand cut French fries, and mayonnaise were "bad." Federal food guidance makes no distinction between eating that steak in 10 minutes in front of the television or eating that steak with friends and family at a celebration. The USDA's discourse of quantification cannot address the goodness of the steak if it had come from a neighbor's farm, if the cow had been grass fed, or if it was dry-aged. A discourse of quantification cannot speak to mayonnaise made from scratch with fresh eggs, extra-virgin olive oil, and just a hint of mustard. A discourse of quantification can count the meal's fat grams, calories, vitamins, and minerals, but it cannot address how a meal tastes or the experience of eating it. This chapter explores discourses with which we can articulate a sense of taste for that steak, apple, or other food using qualitative terms that draw their authority from history, geography, or personal experience.

The language employed by the USDA reveals its commitment to the notion that food is human fuel, and that food serves nutritional functions and avails itself, and the American eater, to measurement, normalization, and standards. In nutrition policy, a discourse of quantification remains the singular voice that exhorts certain eating practices over others. But as this discourse attempts to direct and change the eating patterns of America, other discourses of food exist and grow. These discourses form the foundation for alternative epistemologies of quality. Here I have chosen to examine three alternative discourses that offer the possibility of grounding qualitative knowledge of food in a discourse of taste instead of quantification.

These alternative discourses attempt to define quality using a subjective understanding of food. As such, these discourses provide an eater with alternative ways of describing and knowing "good" and "bad" food. Discourses of taste, ones in which individuals are the arbiters of quality, empower eaters with the ability to judge a food based on their own experience of eating. These qualitative discourses draw their authority from disciplines and sentiments different from science. A discourse of taste that issues from the authority of history might cast quality in terms of tradition or techniques for making food taste a particular way in order to preserve culture or ritual. A discourse of taste that issues from geography might attend to quality by highlighting the idiosyncrasies and particularities of a region's food, the authority of which comes from difference and not normalization. A discourse of taste that issues from personal experience is grounded in the pleasure of eating in particular ways, at particular times, and with particular people. These discourses supplement and complement a discourse of quantification and provide different authoritative grounds upon which to build an epistemology of quality. Thus, this chapter explores alternative ways to communicate food, how to eat, and notions of quality.

The goal of elucidating these alternatives is manifold. These other discourses provide a set of tools with which to see the shortcomings of a discourse of quantification and the policies of the USDA. My hope is that one may be able to use these discourses to examine, or reflect upon, some of the current problems with food and eating in America. I do not wish to cast a discourse of quantification, science, or its methods as villains, or as causes of the current public health crises. I wish only to acknowledge alternative ways of talking about food, and consider them in the context of enumerated food as possible epistemological alternatives. Discourses of taste deriving authority from history, geography, or experience are an alternative form of communication with radically different ends than a discourse of quantification. Each of the three discourses I address assumes an authoritative voice, but does not use science as the defining epistemological feature of qualitative judgments. The authority is the eater, the farmer, the chef, or the gastronome.

It is not my intention to locate *all* possible alternatives to a discourse of quantification. Because alternative discourses reside in diverse places, and frequently lack official or institutional status, identifying all alternative discourses would be impossible. This chapter provides a set of rhetorical themes that will help identify and analyze discourses of food. These analytical tools serve five functions. First, these tools will help point to where alternative food discourses reside. Second, such tools provide the grounds for a critical approach to USDA and food policy founded on a distinctly different language. Third, such discourses provide the opportunity to reconstruct the importance of taste, experience, tradition, and location—all concepts that a discourse of quantification does not, and cannot, account for. Fourth, such discourses supplement a discourse of quantification by offering a more complete picture of the human and subjective processes of eating, and perhaps even a broader understanding of quality. And fifth, such discourses can help explain why the USDA has failed to promote public health. I do not intend to offer a historical account of the origin of such discourses. I understand that what follows may be an impoverished version of history. However, this chapter aims to be functional and constructive. The examples I choose offer useful suggestions, hints for further work, or starting points for lines of thinking that supplement a quantitative understanding of food. These examples are explicit about their preferred manner of communication, and they are explicit about seeing food as a vehicle for tasty experiences and pleasure. It is for this reason that I respond to a historical problem with contemporary solutions.

These analytic tools emerge from observation in lieu of an externally imposed theoretical structure. In other words, my selection of these texts is guided generally by whether or not the text itself claims to be interested in the pursuit of quality food. Discourses of taste rely on the plurality of many voices, voices that reside and resonate in many resources for communication about food. Within the vast genre of food communication, I have selected cookbooks, food writing, websites, television shows, and newspaper articles that I believe offer the most useful analytic tools. By useful I mean these examples possess terms, techniques, or perspectives that provide the reader with the most powerful bases for considering an alternative understanding of food. My reading of each illustrates the usefulness of the examples.

To accommodate the plurality of voices concerning quality, this chapter is organized around three themes. First, I examine discourses that issue from the authority of history. Such discourses treat food as traditional, ritualistic, and cultural and attempt to pass down knowledge and qualitative understandings of food through techniques of preparation, memory, and menu selection. This discourse of taste aims to preserve instead of invent language and make knowledge claims about quality through referencing tradition and history. Second, I examine discourses that issue from the authority of geography. These discourses contrast the normalizing effects of a discourse of quantification because they point out the impossibility of making generalizations about food when a food's qualities rely on, and embody, the place it comes from. The authority of this discourse derives from particularities in soil, weather, location, and seasons. This discourse is especially pronounced in identifying regional qualities of wine and cheese, or when making arguments for buying food that is seasonal or local. What makes a food "good" by geographical standards is that it maintains an environmental fidelity to its place of origin. Third, I explore a discourse of taste that issues from the authority of experience. This discourse arises organically during conversation and human communication, it is codified in food writing, restaurant reviews, websites, and more recently, the emergence of the social movement Slow Food. These media are dedicated to educating and advocating for the authority of the senses. Knowing the constitution of "good" food relies on partaking in discussions and sharing personal experiences of how a food tastes. Because tastes are individual, this discourse eschews the replacement of personal judgments with measurements and rejects the objectivity of a quantitative discourse. In a discourse of taste, food is "good" because it makes you feel good, and it nourishes the body in immeasurable and sensory ways. This discourse encourages the eater to articulate the experience of their food as something more than calories, energy, or means to bodily function. A discourse of taste attends to human experience, makes the eater the sensory authority, and provides her with a space to articulate her experience and share it with others.

Language and forms of communication that result from history, geography, and experience form the foundation for what can loosely be called discourses of taste. I say loosely here because while a discourse of quantification is clearly located in the media of the USDA, discourses of taste rely on a large variety of mechanisms of communication, lack any coherent or central organization for the control and dissemination of a language, and do not seek hegemonic status in official food policies. Often, I refer to discourses of taste in the plural because there are many voices that contribute words, symbols, and meanings without attempting to develop a single absolute language. Within these discourses are various themes that ground an epistemology of quality. In discourses that issue from history, geography, and experience, taste becomes the arbiter of quality. Although taste implicitly points to the subjectivity of eating, questions of epistemology are still central in such a discourse. Such an epistemology allows us to know quality based on what has been good in the past, what is good in a particular place, and what makes us feel good and elicits pleasure.

Furthermore, the work in this chapter builds on the burgeoning field of food studies. In some ways, this field of study is as old as anthropology. Early anthropologists studied food because of its importance to many cultures (Richards, 1932; Firth, 1934; Du Bois, 1941; and Fortes and Fortes, 1936). More contemporary scholars, building on the connection between culture and foodways, have used symbolic, materialist, and ecological methodologies to explain patterns of food selection and eating practices. As such, the field of food studies has produced a number of ethnographies that demonstrate how food is integrated into culture (Meigs, 1984; Kahn, 1986; Weismantel, 1988; Pollock, 1992; and Dettwyler, 1994). This work explores the ways in which food can be seen as a matrix through which innumerable aspects of life come to intersect, including the mixing, congealing, and dispersing of the sense of cultural and personal identity. Food studies scholars often ask the following questions: how can food have different meanings and uses for different people? What role does food play in constituting cultural traditions and beliefs? How does food function to foster community feeling or drive wedges between people? How do people use food to define themselves as individuals, groups, or whole societies? How do biological constraints shape our eating habits? How have biology and culture interacted through eating practices and farming and distribution techniques? Obviously such questions are distinctly different than the kinds of questions that the USDA continues to ask (Telfer, 1996; Counihan and Esterik, 1997; Visser, 1995; Villas, 1982; Curtin and Heldke, 1992; Lupton, 1996). In addition, food studies scholarship investigates issues in food policy, food distribution, agricultural science, and applied nutrition all from the perspectives of economics, history, anthropology, geography, psychology, history, literature, and film studies. The notion of quality food, therefore, can be pursued from a larger variety of perspectives and is not simply reduced to a discourse of quantification.

In this particular chapter, I do not follow the methodologies of anthropologists or sociologists, those working in the mainstream of food studies. Instead, as a rhetorician, I am interested in the ways in which specific ways of talking about food ground, legitimize, or authorize specific claims. From the perspective of communication, the question becomes: why do we believe one thing is true and not another? In other words, why are certain justifications of eating practices or descriptions of food particularly persuasive? Accordingly, I argue that a discourse of quantification is not the only way to generate authoritative claims, and that other kinds of discourse generate authority and ground knowledge claims in other kinds of ways. This chapter, therefore, makes a descriptive argument in that I claim that the language of science and numbers is not the only way to generate knowledge, and a theoretical argument that attempts to explain how and why some of these other discourses are able to generate authority and legitimate knowledge claims. I am indebted to the growing field of food studies, but I hope to extend some of that work through careful attention to language. Moreover, this chapter hopes to open the question of whether or not American foodways (and here I use "American" to signify the construction of a national identity) will continue to be controlled by a discourse or quantification or whether there are viable alternatives with other forms of language capable of carrying the burden of distinguishing good food from bad.

Discourses of Taste and the Authority of History

Discourses that issue from the authority of history differ from a discourse of quantification in important ways. Discourses of history aim to preserve old ways of food communication, and in lieu of inventing new words to describe food, techniques, and eating, it aims to uphold a language that relies on the authority of past experience. Cookbooks, food magazines, and food writing that highlight tradition all attempt to tie people to past experiences in order to preserve a way of talking about food that encourages eaters to use their history as a guide for what to eat. A historical discourse aims to pass down knowledge of food that is both practical as well as ritualistic. Such a discourse differs from a discourse rooted in science, because its rationales for eating are based not on nutrition, but custom, techniques, and practices, all of which rejoice in the social functions of food, as well as its taste.

Cookbooks, in particular ones that highlight techniques of certain well-established cuisines, use history to explain why to cook in a particular way, and to establish an alternative epistemology of quality.[1] In *Essentials of Classic Italian Cooking*, Marcella Hazan (2000) writes:

> Both the revised and the newly added recipes in this book move on the same track, in pursuit not of novelty, but of taste. The taste they have been devised to achieve wants not to astonish, but to reassure. It issues from the cultural memory, the enduring world of generations of Italian cooks, each generation setting a place at table where the next one can feel at ease and at home. It is a pattern of cooking that can accommodate improvisations and fresh intuitions . . . as long as it continues to be a pattern we can recognize, as long as its evolving forms comfort us with that essential attribute of the civilized family life, familiarity. (p. xi)

For Hazan, food that tastes good comes from recognition and reassurance, and it is history that serves as the authoritative and epistemological voice. In her book she attempts to pass on knowledge of what works in the kitchen, but also to highlight the contribution familiarity and "cultural memory" make to the understanding of quality. Hazan recognizes that "improvisations" and "intuitions," modern inventions and iterations of traditional foods, are bound to arise, but while they may taste just as good, the acceptance of these inventions comes from their resemblance to the past. According to Hazan, taste is made up of myriad components, it remains constant in the "enduring world of generations of Italian cooks," and it relies on personal recollection to educe pleasure. Here, good taste issues from remembering the feeling of being "at home," a feeling that cannot be captured by measurement. Knowledge of quality for Hazan cannot be reduced to an exact standard of good or bad, because the determination of quality is as idiosyncratic as each family history. It is memory that authorizes and legitimates specific claims about quality, and it is the articulation and explanation of those memories within cookbooks like Hazan's that does the rhetorical work of grounding a discourse of taste.

The purpose of the cookbook for Hazan is to follow "the whole course of transmitted skills and intuitions in homes throughout the Italian peninsula and the islands" (p. 5). Whether it is "aristocrat's homes, merchant's homes, peasant's homes," tradition or history is tied to and learned through family life. Hazan claims that "there is no such thing as Italian *haute cuisine* because there are no high or low roads in Italian cooking." If, as Hazan says, "all roads lead to the home," then the home becomes the site for the transmission of history and the development of a language of tradition. In fact understanding home traditions and family histories are the defining characteristics of quality Italian cooking. To extend this line of thought, Hazan's philosophy gives us tools for everyone to use in understanding our relationship to food and our evaluations of it. Her use of home as a theme need not be limited to Italian traditions but can apply to everyone in the sense that it offers a space for the sharing of "cultural memory" and the transmission of skills, knowledge, and sentiments that link us to our own past. The cookbook is the rhetorical site for the transmission of this cultural memory and thus is essential in grounding claims about good food.

Following the same line of thought, Julia Child (1966), in *Mastering the Art of French Cooking*, encourages the reader to learn certain well-established cooking techniques and traditional dishes. The reward for learning these techniques is the immeasurable success: taste.

> All of the techniques employed in French cooking are aimed at one goal: how does it taste? The French are seldom interested in unusual combinations or surprise presentations. With an enormous background of traditional dishes to choose from, the Frenchman takes his greatest pleasure from a well-known dish impeccably cooked and served. (p. viii)

Here, Child points out that taste, above all, is the greatest attribute a food can have, and one from which the eater derives the "greatest pleasure." Child relies on the authority of proven techniques, and "well-known" dishes that are a pleasure to eat, to define good food. Child's cookbook discursively captures the essences of these well-known techniques and dishes so as to preserve their rhetorical importance in the maintenance of culture.

In addition to crafting alternative criteria for good food using a discourse incommensurable with a discourse of quantification, Child also crafts criteria for what makes a good cook or a conscientious eater. A good cook masters the techniques for making food *taste* good, and a good eater has the ability to identify food from which he can derive *pleasure*. The good eater or good cook assesses herself using a language of taste issuing from personal history. We can assess good food by how it was tastefully prepared in the past, so that it may be good in the future. Thus, the good cook acknowledges a food's history and uses it as a basis for her understanding of "good" in the future. A good eater assesses food using his pleasure and palate as a guide, and crafts a personal understanding of good by hearkening back to other eating occasions and remembering individual sensations and experiences. Whether the eater had been to France or eaten French cuisine does not matter to Child. Instead her rationale for crafting an understanding of food through engaging with *Mastering the Art of French Cooking* is historical, and a history manifested in taste. The past provides the rhetorical grounds on which to make qualitative judgments.

It is useful to compare the cooking techniques that aim to accomplish a tasty dish discussed by Child with the techniques of scientists in the laboratory. Wilbur Atwater used the calorimeter in pursuit of new knowledge, and thus invented techniques in his scientific laboratory that performed two functions. First, out of a dissatisfaction with current and past ways of understanding food, Atwater's scientific practice invented methods to produce new ways of understanding and ultimately new ways of describing food. Second, in pursuing new knowledge about food, the scientific practices broke foods down to analyze their constituent parts. The goal of Child's work (as well as many other cookbook authors) is precisely the opposite. The cooking practices she offers are meant to preserve the past, and are meant to build knowledge from what already exists. The calorimeter's treatment of food, burning it until nothing but an ashy residue remains, represents the manner in which scientific techniques strip away the human elements of food in pursuit of new knowledge. In comparison, when Child describes a traditional dish, for example Poulet Rôti, the oven, as an apparatus, is used to constructive rather than destructive ends. For Child, the purpose of the oven is to create "a juicy, brown, buttery, crisp-skinned, heavenly bird," and to do so requires one to "hover over the bird, listen to it, above all see that it is continually basted, and that it is done just to the proper turn" (Child, 1966, p. 240). Learning the skills and techniques defined by Child allows the reader to proactively carry forth his history into the future. As an analytic tool, traditional cooking techniques are a mechanism for preserving quality and supplement certain numerated and scientific kitchen practices like exact measurements or baking temperatures.[2] These quantitative techniques ought not to be replaced but should be the grounds for establishing continuity with the past.

The importance of carrying traditions forward is not limited to the perceived haute cuisine of France. In *My Mexico*, Diana Kennedy (1998) describes recipes that have long held an important place in Mexican culture:

> And the more I travel, the more I realize that most families, even in the smallest communities, have a culinary history: recipes and methods handed down from one generation to another. If all this had been recorded over the years, it would reveal a lot about the changes in these societies through good times and bad, changes in climate and therefore agriculture, and the effects of political and social influences brought about by workers coming and going between the larger cities and the United States. (p. vi–vii)

Here, Kennedy uses the themes of home, history, and tradition as mechanisms for understanding politics, economics, and environmental issues. Recorded traditional recipes provide more than just a means to produce good food. Each recipe in Kennedy's book begins with a short anecdote on the origin of the dish, usually involving a specific person, family, or place. Telling these stories creates a context for understanding the development and importance of specific dishes as well as their relationship to larger socioeconomic factors. Here the history of food becomes a valuable resource for understanding transformations in society and for providing future generations with tools for understanding their past, with a "wealth of culinary knowledge and folklore," and with "fascinating human stories." These contribute to making food "a language all its own that transcends mere words or actions" (p. ix). Here food itself can be used as a means of rhetorical invention, and it is a form of rhetorical invention authorized by the past.

By understanding food as a language capable of passing on knowledge and history, Kennedy recounts what food can symbolize beyond nourishment: "I am always urging cooks I meet to write down (if they can write) the basics of their recipes and demonstrate them to a younger member of the family who can take more detailed notes, so that this knowledge is not lost in the changes that are beginning to infiltrate, and that I fear will invade, Mexico" (p. vii). Preserving taste, techniques, and natural ingredients, therefore, becomes a way to preserve Mexican history itself, and the celebration of that history at the table provides the means for resisting the invasion of an American ideology.[3] Traditions are worthy of preservation because they create good food and leave a discursive residue for understanding a culture, in all of its lived experience. In this way, historical accounts of eating work in opposition to a discourse of quantification, which tries to eliminate cultural identity in favor of universal standards of measurement.

Many food studies scholars have studied cookbooks in order to determine the ways in which these media of communication figure health, purity, identity, and culture. Sometimes recipes can be read as a code for deeper cultural meaning, or as an embedded discourse signifying a variety of social relationships and gendered norms, or as a narrative that engages the reader/cook in a larger conversation about culture and history (Floyd and Forster, 2003). In each of these iterations, the recipe is open to subjective intervention and interpretation, and is thus categorically distinct from USDA-sanctioned food guides. Food studies scholarship has also traced the changing role of recipes depending on historical context. For example, Valerie Mars (1994) writes about upper-class Victorian children eating only blandly favored foodstuffs for fear of stimulating their appetites. Laura Shapiro (2001) has written about the cooking classes of the late nineteenth-century domestic science movement and the attempt to enforce an "American" cuisine over against anything considered "foreign." Feminist scholars have attempted to recover recipe writing as an example of creativity and the construction of community (Leonardi, 1989). Some argue that women are empowered by their relationship to food, as embodied in cookbooks (Theophano, 2002). This variety of ways of reading cookbooks signals the subjectivity of the discourses at work within those books. However, as Janet Floyd and Laurel Forster contend, "cookery writing is indeed frequently involved in the work of imaginatively recreating the past. . . . Personal histories or pasts, constructed through memory, or the process of remembering with others, are often centered on food" (2003, p. 7). This form of "heightened memory" for Floyd and Forster implicates the senses in a historical narrative. It is often this appeal to history that authorizes and legitimizes the claims made within cookbooks.

The three cookbooks I have mentioned, therefore, can be seen as part of a larger discursive trend explicitly committed to preserving traditional cuisines. Cookbook authors like Madhur Jaffrey whose specialty is Indian cuisine, or Joan Nathan who traces recipes of the Jewish faith, use history as the inspiration for their texts and as the rhetorical means for communicating taste. These authors offer audiences, who may or may not be part of the cultural tradition these books refer to, the means for making food that tastes good in light of the authority of history. These books, and ones with similar goals, are not specific prescriptions for how or what to eat. Unlike a discourse of quantification, discourses of taste arising from history celebrate the familiarity of iterations on specific themes. While they admit variations in methods, techniques, and histories, the purpose of these books is to offer readers proven criteria for judging quality, criteria that have made up significant and meaningful parts of a particular culture's past. Most importantly, these cookbooks produce a plurality of discourses of taste, none of which seek singular or definitive authority on questions of quality. In other words, Madhur Jaffrey does not claim that Indian cooking is superior to Italian cooking or even that one Indian province's cooking is superior to another. The tradition that Jaffrey celebrates is specific, localized, and grounded in particular methods that are authoritative in their own terms, and are accessible to a variety of audiences without claiming hegemonic status as the sole arbiter of quality. The history passed down in cookbooks is a useful tool for judging quality, for learning cooking techniques, and for understanding the origins of taste.

Cookbooks are not the only discursive space for celebrating the importance of tradition and history. Frequently, food magazines contextualize food using historical narratives. These magazines include recipes and feature articles that describe the context of a food that might include a description of its place of origin, its growers or creators, its role in history or the development of its place in a particular diet. All of these factors encourage a different set of criteria from which to judge a food's quality. Even media that use a discourse of quantification to justify their publication, like *Cooking Light* or *Weight Watchers* magazines (which rely on the reader being savvy about the scientific functions and language of food), uses context to encourage the reader to eat in a particular way that supplements a data-laden approach.

Food magazines often group food by social not physiological function. The reader then gets a different sense of the context of the food and a different definition of "good." A *Saveur* article on green peppers reads:

> My California grandmother had great green pepper moves. Even in the summer, with only a couple of fans to ease the searing Sacramento heat, she'd fire up the oven to make stuffed ones—because my grandfather loved them, and hers were a sublime expression of love. The stuffing and the glaze were delicious, but it was the soft, leathery pepper flesh, with its grassy-green flavor, that really made that dish. Even today, I can close my eyes and taste it. (Hirsheimer, 2000, p. 90)

For the author, his knowledge of quality green peppers arises from his past. His personal history, where he was, who he was with, and what time of year it was, all color his perception of the vegetable. The author uses food to identify a moment in time, and that particular food transports him to that moment. The author's description of "delicious" comes from recreating the past, and he articulates taste using language that captures a historical moment.

In each issue of the food magazine *Saveur*, a section is dedicated to celebrating a "Classic" food or recipe. According to the editor, "because we approach food in context, as something intimately connected to geography, history and everyday life, we can't help being aware of the political and social conditions that surround its production, preparation and consumption" (Kalins, 1997, p. 16). By addressing foods that have had their gastronomic heyday or have become retro chic, the Classic section teaches the reader how to cook a particular dish or food, the origins of that food, and illustrates the significance of it. For example, the September/October 2002 issue presents a recipe for challah bread and an account of the role of challah bread in Jewish culture. When the author "learned about its [challah bread] history and religious significance" that "soft, crusty bread" became a pleasurable experience, a connection to her "Brooklyn home on Friday night," and part of a "bread-making tradition" (Goldberg, p. 41). This Classic column teaches the reader that the taste of a food can bring one back home and bring one back into a 2000-year-old tradition signifying the 12 tribes of Israel. It is impossible to quantify challah bread's role in this enduring culture, and thus challah bread offers the reader a reconstructed understanding of quality. More importantly, the rhetorical effects of recounting that history position the reader within a particular cultural tradition and thus ties taste to that tradition.

For the past 62 years, the food magazine *Gourmet* dedicates an entire issue to the foods and practices of American Thanksgiving. Perhaps more than any other holiday, Thanksgiving in America is tied most closely to food and eating. According to Ruth Reichl, the editor of *Gourmet*, "by asking the question—what does your family eat at Thanksgiving?" food historian Ian Dengler could reconstruct anyone's personal history (1999, p. 28). Dengler claims to be able to tell where a person is from in the United States, her cultural heritage, and how long her family has been in America simply by knowing what she eats for Thanksgiving. *Gourmet* marks these cultural tweaks of the American tradition by offering a variety of recipes each year. And the recipes always continue the line of thought that "Americans sit down to the same turkey dinner, but each family actually makes the meal its own" (p. 28). In other words, cooking "is a way of connecting with the past—and a promise to the future" (Reichl, 2001, p. 18). Unlike traditional cookbooks, *Gourmet* offers new recipes and new techniques (like recently popularized turkey brining and frying), but like traditional cookbooks, the significance of the dishes derives from their recognition as a time-honored part of the Thanksgiving meal.

Food magazines also highlight the culinary aspects of more common American life. *Bon Appetit* looks to the tradition of Sunday football as a setting for certain foods and conviviality. For the author of "For Super Bowl, a Super Party," foods that perhaps may seem ordinary—tuna sandwiches and grilled sausage—hearken back to the family gathering and particular techniques of preparation. For example, during football games the author's father was "so meticulous in the way he squished around the tuna and mayo and how he slashed and grilled those wursts and served them up with Boston baked beans" (Gold, 2003, p. 43). A summer issue of *Saveur* uses the backdrop of the Iowa State Fair as the context for a recipe for corn dogs: "The corn dog has become the very symbol of the Fair's pork-centered, corn-crusted, deep fried soul. 'Corn dog,' says longtime fairgoer Arlene Eckhart, '*is* the Fair' " (Eskin, 1998, p. 45). This is an example of a linguistic association far different than the one achieved by Atwater with the calorie. Food here is linked to traditions beyond the food itself and those traditions are what give the food its meaning (instead of the food's hidden properties). Rhetorically, this way of generating meeting allows one to ground qualitative judgments on these cultural factors and not on scientific factors.

These examples show that personal, family, and community histories act as an authority for determining good food. Defining "traditional" foods need not be located in 2000-year-old religious customs or marked by significant historical events. The significance of discourses of taste that the tuna sandwich or the corn dog illustrate is that the ability to practice a technique or further a history can be found in families gathering around the television or attending a local fair. In these instances, the identification and definition of quality food becomes part of living in a local, community-centered tradition, and imparts authority to the common person by virtue of their participation in family or community rituals.

By referencing history, communication about food seeks to transmit techniques, feelings, and traditions that connect an eater to family members, to larger communities, or to a common cultural heritage. Such a language does not seek to categorize eaters or control eating habits with standards invented by science, but instead respects individuality and idiosyncrasy as variations on common themes that add to our understanding of taste. The act of transmitting knowledge about taste and quality requires a language that is distinctive, yet shared and common—a language open to interpretation based on the subjectivity of taste but in line with the themes that have conditioned the possibility for tasty food in the past. Such a language offers tools to understand why we eat in the manner we do, what foods find their way onto our table, and what techniques are best employed in cooking. More importantly, however, such a language provides tools for a broader understanding of our relationship to food. This understanding, and the acknowledgment of themes like home, tradition, or technique can be used in critiquing USDA food guides, in continuing traditions of excellence, and in supplementing scientific approaches to food. By preserving traditional descriptions of food, and by locating questions of judgment in the person who possesses knowledge of the past, a language of food that issues from history points to the possibility of constructing a valuable and valid conception of taste outside of a discourse of quantification. Food can symbolize something other than its physiological function. The authority of history aims to establish an understanding of food that highlights this possibility and offers well-established means for developing an understanding of food that symbolizes more than nutrients, calories, or serving sizes.

Discourses of Taste and the Authority of Geography

Discourses of taste that issue from history are complemented by, and often tied closely to, geography or place. Cultural traditions are established equally by the particular foods grown in a region, as they are by the techniques passed down from generation to generation. French food, Italian food, Indian food, and even American food are almost always associated with the land that produces the food available for eating. In fact variations of traditions are often derived from variations in geography, sometimes even within a particular country.[4] The land, therefore, becomes an authoritative factor in deciding what to eat, when to eat it, and what tastes good.

For example, wine is closely associated with and defined by geography. French wines are identified by their *Appellation d'Origine Contrôlée*, a moniker that designates the region in which the grapes were grown and indicates that the grapes have been processed in a certain way that ensures a certain product's taste. That this information is vital to knowing wine demonstrates an alternative approach to an epistemology of quality. Knowing a wine's origin is essential in identifying qualities of its taste, more so than the number of calories, or even its purported healthy role in a "good" diet. Geography then, becomes fundamental in the act of naming and knowing wine. In fact, the geography of wine naming is so important that the governments of Italy and France regulate the process and require labels to adhere to explicit standards.[5] Because a wine's origin is a factor upon which to judge its "goodness," authority regarding questions of taste derives from place or region.

It is useful to compare the FDA's Nutrition Labeling Education Act with the *Appellation d'Origine Contrôlée* designation of France. While the former agency uses labels to identify the same scientific properties in foods, the latter uses labels to identify the differences between wines. The goal of the NLEA is to use a standard set of scientific terms that allow the consumer to compare different foods and make judgments about quality based on the common quantities that different foods share. The NLEA generalizes food across regions, seasons, and types. In contrast, the *appellation contrôlée* designation of wines points to the impossibility of comparing different comestibles with a single set of criteria. A specific geographical label renders a wine unique and prevents that wine from being easily compared to other wines from different regions. Questions of quality, then, occur at the level of the eccentricity of each winemaker from each *appellation*. The wine drinker uses geography to distinguish grapes and flavors, and vineyards and vintages to determine taste.

The French concept of *appellation contrôlée* is built on the notion of *terroir*. Hugh Johnson (1999) defines *terroir* as "a French word meaning soil and site in the ecological totality. A wine is said to have *un goût de terroir* (a taste of the soil) when it has gathered certain nuances of taste and flavor from the land on which it was produced" (p. 114). According to Johnson "a Frenchman will tell you it [*terroir*] matters most of all" in deciding a wine's quality. This concept implicates the geology of the soil in which grapes are grown, as well as "the topography of the vineyard, the climate of the surrounding area, the amount of sunlight the vineyard receives and other natural factors" (Bastianich and Lynch, 2002, p. viii). These factors affect the "personalities" of different wines. Based on the concept of *terroir*, claims, judgments, and knowledge about wine all issue from an intimate understanding of place. Certain grapes and wines thrive in certain *terroirs* and thus derive their tastes and sensations, as well as their quality, from location. Andrew Jefford (2000) writes about the French geographical *appellations* of St. Emilion and Pomerol:

> Merlot [grapes] dominates Bordeaux's right bank, most celebratedly in St. Emilion and Pomerol. The lushness and soft, sensual warmth of the best Pomerols and the aromatic meatiness of the best St. Emilions have made them the darlings of the wine world. This, in turn, has sent Merlot racing around the new vineyards of both hemispheres as growers attempt to reproduce those winning characteristics—not, so far, with great success. (p. 26)

The failure of the winegrowers' attempts to reproduce the success of the Merlot grape in "Bordeaux's right bank" in other parts of the world illustrates the role *terroir* plays in crafting a wine's "personality." The attempts to reproduce the unique flavors and sensations that the Merlot grapes derive from the sunlight in St. Emilion, or the hilliness of Pomerol, are destined to fail. Unlike a scientific laboratory, where conditions can be controlled, and sunlight may be measured in lumens and simulated with fluorescent bulbs, geographic characteristics of a certain region, and even the practices of certain winemakers make successful wine growing difficult to measure—sometimes it is more a question of art than science.

Robert Parker Jr., "the biggest critic in the world" of wine, argues that the primary function of the winemaker is to "let the *terroir* express itself" (McInerny, 2002, pp. 169–170). Parker goes so far as to claim that his "legacy" as a wine critic is built upon the premise of identifying and understanding the concept of *terroir* in wine making. And he is not alone. Jay McInerny (2002) argues that Andre Tchelistcheff, one of the founding winemakers in Napa Valley, California, "was among the first to import the French concept of *terroir* to the valley; hundreds of years of grape growing had allowed the French to parse the viticultural landscape into hundreds of regions and subregions based on nuances of soil type and microclimate. Tchelistcheff attempted to do something similar in Napa" (p. 174). In wine drinking and wine making, the language used must always refer to the place from which the wine comes. Geography then, has an authoritative voice in directing practices, in knowing and tasting wine. Rhetorically, the effect of the use of the concept of *terroir* is to build an association with the context in which wine is grown. Unlike the calorie (that mysterious and invisible quality of food), *terroir* both literally and figuratively grounds the quality of wine in the characteristics of the soil, and the characteristics of the soil legitimate the claims that are made about particular wines.

In the case of wine, geography obviously opens questions of place, but geography can also ask questions of timing. The seasons change and with those changes, the food available from the soil changes as well. Seasonality is as much a question of geography as *terroir*. In addition, seasonality forces the eater to acknowledge "localness" as a tool for judging the quality of a food. Using these criteria, when a food comes from nearby and is made available for consumption soon after it is harvested, it is of a higher quality than food that has been shipped from thousands of miles away, and whose ripening process has been controlled off the vine, or out of the soil. Different regions have different growing seasons, each yielding unique and particular foods. In this regard, quality food is a function of both the time of year and the place it grows. The themes of seasonality and locality are useful for understanding how geography can be a determining factor in taste.

It is often the case that cookbooks and food writing use seasons to guide when to eat what foods.[6] Pellegrino Artusi (1996) offers monthly menus along with the following advice:

Let your market and the weather dictate your menu. Use only the freshest ingredients—ingredients that look tired will taste tired, and are not worth the trouble. If the weather is cold, you will want something substantial to keep the chill at bay. Lighter foods work better in the summer. (p. 473)

In order to follow Artusi's advice about the "freshest ingredients" one must understand their local geography and let it dictate what foods will be available at certain times of the year. This involves identifying both the moment at which the ingredients are at their freshest and the general time periods during which foods are harvested. Both of these concerns, with the utmost freshness and peak harvest times, are further subject to geographic idiosyncrasies and can even change from year to year. Thus, one must remain attentive to shifts in weather patterns or climate, and be able to judge the effects of these shifts on the food growing in a region. Language that issues from claims to seasonality and geography provide discursive tools to critique food that is substandard. Foods that are not from the local "market," or do not respect the patterns of the weather, are not as "good."

Farmers' markets remain an essential space for learning about a region's edible bounty. Such markets are always tied to the land and to the seasons, and therefore offer the farmer and customer an opportunity to engage in dialogue about the freshness or the quality of the food for sale. The farmer can thus introduce new ways to describe flavors, tastes, and knowledge to those who may not be as intimately associated with the land. American soul food chef Edna Lewis (1988) pays tribute to the role of the farmers' market as an authority regarding issues of taste:

If you eat a vegetable when it has been grown under the right conditions, including reaching maturity at the right time of year, it tastes as good as can be. I think it is important to keep this in mind—which is why I am delighted that so many cities have established farmers' markets where local farmers can sell their produce. (pp. 6–7)

For Lewis, understanding the seasons and communicating with farmers results in food tasting "as good as can be."

Today, nearly 3,000 farmers' markets across the United States provide a vital space for the exploration of fresh, local food, while just 25 years ago, only a handful of such markets existed. Leslie Brenner (2000) calls this "the biggest change in American gastronomy in the last forty years" (p. 279). "Freshness" is the reason this change is so important to Brenner—"freshness" becomes a guarantee of quality. Deborah Madison (2002) wrote *Local Flavors: Cooking and Eating from America's Farmers' Markets* to pay tribute to both the importance of geography in eating and the value of the local market. "Pride in one's work and one's land," according to Madison, are necessary for keeping farming traditions alive, providing communities with good food, and creating healthy communities" (p. xiii). The farmers' market is *the* place "where we can find food that is impeccably fresh and delicious, truly local and therefore truly seasonal," and the most "sustainable" political and social conditions for understanding quality (p. xvii). Here, the concept of quality transcends taste and encompasses everyday life practices, many of which are implicated by food choices. References to the local and seasonal are the primary grounds on which to base criticisms of standardization at the forefront of the food industry and the science of nutrition. In other words, the authority of geography is a persuasive mechanism for refuting arguments that are rooted in unwavering scientific principles and political and economic thrusts to efficiency. While a tomato may contain scientifically valuable lycopenes, eating a tomato in January in the American northeast all but guarantees a mealy, watery, and flavorless fruit, one that has been harvested before its time and artificially ripened using ethylene gas. Freshness authorizes and legitimizes claims to quality food, and thus the farmers' market, by reestablishing the connection between food and land, rhetorically builds an alternative way of making judgments about good food (a way that privileges the local because of the importance of the land in producing food).

In the restaurant industry, Chef Alice Waters has pioneered and mobilized a discourse of taste founded on geography. In some ways, Waters's restaurant Chez Panisse, and others that ascribe to Waters's philosophy, can be contrasted with the ubiquity and familiarity of McDonald's. While Waters's restaurant focuses on seasonal foods from near by, and has a menu that changes daily, McDonald's provides a standard menu that prides itself on the repeatability of taste around the globe. In the fall and winter, when the colder weather inhibits the growth of new vegetables and the desire for light, chilled foods, Chez Panisse serves warm, heavier soups and stews flavored with mushrooms, beans, and hard-skinned squashes that keep in a cool larder. In the spring and summer Waters serves palate-cleansing fresh salads, grilled vegetables and fish, and fresh fruit. Waters's philosophy also works in opposition to North American grocery stores that pride themselves on the ability to provide all fruits and vegetables all year long. According to Waters, "a good kitchen respects its sources, chooses ingredients that are sound, seasonal, local when possible, and appropriate to the event."[7]

Waters's commitment to encouraging the respect of the seasons and the consumption of local products extends beyond her restaurant. In her Edible Schoolyard project, Waters uses a discourse of taste and the authority of geography to form a foundation for an experiential understanding of food among public school students. In this pilot program in Berkeley, California, middle school students worked with Waters to convert an empty lot into a green space to grow fruits and vegetables. In the Edible Schoolyard, students planted seeds, monitored weather and plant growth, fertilized and harvested. Waters's mission for the garden is to have students develop a sense for the land, and to use that sense to grow food that tastes good. "Our future rests on our being able to take care of our kids and teach them how to take care of the land," Waters said in an interview, "how to nourish themselves, and how to gather at the table" (Bogo, 2002, p. 30).

Waters's philosophy of defining quality in the local has also expanded to operations decidedly downscale. In Quechee, Vermont, the Farmer's Diner has a 50-mile rule for the origin of its ingredients. Farms within 50 miles of the restaurant raise most of the food served there. The Farmer's Diner serves bacon and eggs, blue-plate hamburger specials, and pancakes, a far cry from Waters's warm porcini mushroom salad with Parmesan and curly endive, or her caramelized Bosc pears and crème fraîche ice cream, but the philosophy is the same. The eggs, hamburger meat, bacon, and even the flour for the pancakes, are from local farmers. In the first six months of operation, 70% of the Diner's food budget went to food suppliers in the 50-mile radius. The Farmer's Diner believes that local food is better, politically, environmentally, economically, and gastronomically. Though many of the patrons of the Farmer's Diner may be oblivious to the political and economic ramifications of eating local, they are swayed by the taste: "[owner Tod] Murphy's hamburger, from beef raised on the western side of the Green Mountains in Starksboro [VT], is really, really good" (McKibben, 2003, p. 54). Celebrating the local, and its superior taste, need not be limited to single operations. In and around the Portland, Oregon, region, a chain called Burgerville (with 39 locations) is "devoted to serving dishes that celebrate Northwest ingredients" (Stern and Stern, 2003, p. 54). While the radius for its supplies is larger than the Farmer's Diner, 80% of Burgerville's menu is grown in Washington, Oregon, and Idaho. Burgerville's food focus remains seasonal. Walla-Walla sweet onion rings are available only in the summer months, and the milkshake menu changes seasonally: strawberry shakes in April, blackberry shakes in July, pumpkin shakes in November, and chocolate hazelnut shakes in December.

The rhetorical force of the claim to quality made by such restaurants issues directly from the association of food with the land. It is one's connection to and knowledge of the land that produces quality food.

These considerations of seasonality, localness, and particularity, which draw upon the geographical authority of food, provide alternative approaches to a discourse of quantification. These discourses offer an opportunity to reconstruct the importance of the taste of food in terms of geography and environment. In the instance of wine *appellation* and the concept of *terroir*, a discourse of taste issuing from the authority of geography works in three ways. First, geography becomes a quality of the wine. Just as the calorimeter made numbers a constitutive part of food—something that helped to identify the food, wine *appellation* does the same thing. But the goals of the two systems of classification have different ends. The calorimeter sought to make all food comparable by imparting all food with a requisite set of elements: carbohydrates, fats, and proteins. The designation of an *appellation* or *terroir* seeks to make wines incomparable, and important and distinctive in their own right. This designation of geography orders our relationship to food, but does so using difference and not similarity. Second, the geographic *appellation* can also represent certain qualities of the wine itself and act as a signifier of specific tastes. Wines grown in certain regions have certain distinctive aromas unique to that region, and the interaction of the same grape with different soil may produce radically different taste sensations. A wine from the Crozes-Hermitage region in the Rhone Valley of France may be described as having flavors of "chocolate," "bacon," or "wet hay" (Prial, 2002, F10).[8] But wines made from the same grape varietal (the Syrah), as the Crozes-Hermitage *appellation*, produce very different flavors when planted in Australia or South Africa, perhaps flavors of vanilla or burnt toast or skunk. And third, if we identify a wine by its geography, we allocate certain taste sensations to that geography. If the tastes we experience are pleasant, then geography becomes an arbiter of quality.

Using geography as a tool for assessing the quality of foods places eaters into a unique relationship with their particular locale and allows them to articulate quality in accessible ways. A discourse of taste that relies on these geographic themes makes eaters aware of where they are from, where their food is from, and how the interaction between the two plays an important role in eating. Perhaps the most important discursive aspect of the geographic authority of a discourse of taste is the celebration of the particular and regional. Understanding this aspect of this discourse of taste highlights the extent to which scientific standardization infiltrates the grocery store, chain restaurant menus, and federal nutritional advice. While science and a discourse of quantification encourages and lauds

repeatability and standardization, a discourse of taste celebrates the particularities of food: knowing the farmer who provides the beef for a diner's
chili, eating ripe berries in the summer from a roadside farmers' market,
or learning about which vegetables thrive in local soil. These geographic
particularities outshine the normalizing ability of the language of science
and give individuals a sense of place to their food, a sense that they may
use to judge its quality.

Discourses of Taste and the Authority of Experience

Underlying many discourses of taste, including some that issue from the
authority of history and geography, are discourses that issue from the
authority of experience. These discourses use human practice as the basis
for both crafting and organizing knowledge about quality food. In a
discourse of taste that issues from experience, "good" is defined by personal encounters with food and one's ability to articulate that encounter
to others. Thus, in this discourse of taste, the expert is anyone who eats
and can articulate his or her sentiments about what he or she is eating.
Just as a discourse of quantification can be used to invent language to
organize and order our relationship to food, so too can an experiential
discourse of taste. The emphasis in the latter, however, is the invention of
language that uses pleasure as the organizing principle and privileges the
human sense of taste as arbiter. There are no units with which to measure
the deliciousness of a meal, and there is no way to compare how more
or less tasty one restaurant or food is over another. And so it is in this
discursive realm that a discourse of quantification fails completely. Here,
the epistemology of quality relies on conversation, conviviality, and the
articulation of personal pleasure.

　　In discourses of taste that issues from the authority of experience,
we attempt to *amplify* food experiences and taste and not *reduce* them
as we do with a discourse of quantification. These amplifying discourses
proliferate in spaces that celebrate the sharing of experiences and memories,
the description of those experiences, the universality of the sense of taste,
and the uniqueness of each palate. Websites and blogs, social gatherings
and movements, and radio and television programs about good food and
pleasurable eating experiences all provide fora for the communication of
experience. These locations and the discourses that occupy them provide
an opportunity for the reconstruction of the importance of the subjective
and qualitative aspects of food. Food studies scholarship has been intensely
interested in analyzing and attempting to understand these subjective and
qualitative aspects of experience in philosophical (Curtin and Heldke, 1992;

Telfer, 1996) and sociological (Anderson, 2005; Warde, 1997) terms. My interests are less in the qualities of taste experiences and more in the ways in which those experiences serve as justifications for claims to quality.

Beginning with Duncan Hines (a real person and not just a brand name) in the early 1940s, assessing the quality of a restaurant by eating its food, and often writing a review of that food, has long provided a space for articulating the authority of experience through taste.[9] Reviewers would eat across a restaurant's menu, describe the tastes they experienced, and subsequently determine whether those sensations were pleasurable or not. The reviewer's tools for assessment were the range of flavors available for the palate to experience. The assessments were subsequently articulated using the reviewer's own descriptive language. It was the subjectivity of the tongue that founded this epistemology of quality. Restaurant review resources are now published in book form (like the *Zagat's* or *Time Out* guides), and daily or weekly in newspapers (most major American broadsheet newspapers have a restaurant reviewer) and magazines (the *New Yorker*, for example, runs a weekly restaurant column).[10] Frequently, though, restaurant reviews focus on high-end dining, eating experiences whose quality is assessed using more than just the taste of the food. Good dining establishments pride themselves on having polite waitstaff, an expert wine sommelier, and chic dining room designs. When reviewers attend these restaurants, they frequently make mention of these features, in addition to the food. A *New Yorker* review of the restaurant Capitale reads, "[T]he space is tremendous: nearly an acre of marble, forested with Corinthian columns and Jurassic potted palms. . . . Rounding out the bewildering atmosphere is the music: boomer pop courtesy of satellite radio . . . the waiter, citing popular demand, pushes the rib-eye—the most expensive dish" (Paumgarten, 2003, p. 25). While these kinds of reviews do have elements of gastronomic qualitative discourse, there is a barrier to contributing opinions—these restaurants tend to be expensive and not everyone is a restaurant critic with a circulating newspaper.

Recently, however, websites have provided an electronic forum for eaters to communicate their experience to others. For example, chowhound.com provides a discursive space for both the development of a language of experience and the proliferation of that language through public dissemination.[11] The concept of Chowhound was the brainchild of Jim Leff, whose goal was "to provide a non-hypey haven" where "anyone who eats is welcome to stop by for unbiased, savvy chow advice or just to sit back and watch in amazement." According to the website, self-dubbed Chowhounds "know where the good stuff is, and they never settle for less than optimal deliciousness, whether dining in splanky [sic] splendor, or grabbing a quick slice of pizza."[12] The purpose of the Chowhound site is to allow eaters to share information about restaurants, bakeries, food shops, and recipes. The site is organized by geography, with each region of the United States represented by clickable links. From there, you may click on a region and message boards appear with discussion threads you may join. Alternatively, you may start your own thread and seek information from other Chowhounds.

This site is the epitome of a discourse of taste that draws authority from experience. Contributors write an account of what they ate, a personal definition of "good," and thus an experiential understanding of the epistemology of quality. A December 20, 2003, posting on the Midwest Chowhound message board titled "My Twin Cities Chinese Food Odyssey" reads:

> Well, it has been 6 months since I moved back to the Twin Cities from NYC, where I was born and raised, and since returning I have been on a quest for Chinese food to make me happy. I really like the spicy baked squid at Shuang Cheng; it is quite different from the salted pepper squid I have had elsewhere, more of a 5-spice taste, but still excellent. I have yet to find another dish to draw me there, but I haven't tried the whole fish yet. And I go for the squid frequently. Any additions? Any place with truly great noodles?[13]

This posting received five responses, one respondent claimed: "I'd be curious to know what you think of the salt and pepper squid at Peking Garden on the East Campus of the U . . . I love their squid."[14] Another respondent recommends a restaurant for noodles, and a third adds to this recommendation with a caveat: "I second the recommendation for The Tea House—BUT you must ask for the SESCHUAN [sic] MENU. Otherwise you'll end up eating real bland food intended for non-adventurous Midwesterns [sic]."[15] Here, each Chowhound uses his or her own experiences to build knowledge of good food and a language for describing it. The initial query has crafted a link between her mission for pleasure and good food saying, "I have been on a quest for Chinese food to make me happy." Respondents attempt to aid her mission by providing accounts of their own pleasurable experiences, and advice for how to achieve "good" food. This communication of experiences between eaters crafts an alternative epistemology of quality. Chowhounds seek the advice of others because they have developed their own understanding of "good." In lieu of quantitative terms as markers of "good" and "bad," descriptors like "bland" and "5-spice" become part of a language of quality and necessarily implicate the taste of food in order to make judgment possible. The rhetorical invention and use of such a language is clearly subjective and celebrates that subjectivity. What is interesting is that the more idiosyncratic and creative the description of taste, the more often that description is seen as legitimate. In other words, the creative invention of descriptions of experience authorizes claims to know good food.

A Chowhound posting from the Southwest site titled "Where to find pancetta in Phoenix?" reads: "Have a pasta recipe that I want to try. It's basically just pasta, olive oil, and pancetta, so I want to get really good pancetta. Where can I find it in the Phoenix area?"[16] This thread received several responses, each Chowhound giving an account of his or her favorite place to purchase the cured pork. One reader recommends "AJ's," another "the deli at Alma School and Baseline," and a third reader shares with the posting other possible pleasurable tastes to be had:

> There is an Italian/Greek family deli (they make own sausage) on Dunlap just west of I-17 right before 34th Ave on the left called Romanelli's. They have pancetta, assorted cheeses including ricotta insalata [sic] and fresh mozzarella. If you get there and there are fresh chocolate eclairs do yourself a favor and get one. Crisp on the outside and creamy in the inside. Yum![17]

This pancetta-in-Phoenix thread illustrates the multiple definitions of "good" pancetta. One reader thinks AJ's is the tastiest option, another opts for the deli at Alma School, and a third Romanelli's, epitomizing the fundamentally subjective nature of good taste, and the impossibility of standardizing the experience of food. What is important in chowhound. com is the continuity of conversation. There are no absolute definitions of "good" pancetta, as the taste of pork is unable to be measured, just as there is no end point for determining and defining "good." The discourse of taste is a discourse in flux, constantly changing to accommodate opinion and crafting new ways of talking about and understanding quality food. The foundation of this discourse is the plurality of voices that contribute definitions of "good," and the discourse is enriched by more voices, not one authoritative voice. Communication around taste is always uncertain, ambiguous, and open-ended without the need for finality or transparency. Conversations about taste are messy, like a molten chocolate cake spilling out to the reaches of the plate—the Chowhound website clearly illustrates this.

In contrast to the open-ended dialogue on chowhound.com, the Slow Food movement offers a more organized and politically active attempt to develop a discourse of taste based on experience. The Slow Food movement began in Italy in 1986. Its goal at the outset was to "counter the tide of standardization of taste and the manipulation of consumers around the world."[18] Slow Food meeting groups, or convivia, exist in 83 countries around the world. Each convivium gathers together to celebrate taste and pursue new gastronomic experiences. For example, events held by the Pittsburgh convivium of Slow Food included a balsamic vinegar tasting, wild mushroom foraging expedition, a Neapolitan pizza night, a local cheese tasting, a lamb picnic, a pig roast, and a South Indian themed dinner. These events provide an opportunity for people to meet, taste, and, most importantly, discuss food. Each event allows the members to experience new tastes, compare the tastes with others, and craft their own opinion about what tastes good. The Pittsburgh convivium's events were not duplicated at other Slow Food events in America or around the world. The events were developed because they celebrated the foods that the local region had to offer. The grazing fields of Latrobe, Pennsylvania, where the Jamison family have their lamb farm, allowed the Pittsburgh convivium to taste freshly killed local meat, fed on nearby land, and raised by farmers who explained the process of lamb husbandry to the group. The experience that issues from such events allows for the development of a connection between the eater, the farmer, and the land and thus organizes the experience of eating and tasting in a more specific, educational, and rich manner. In other words, group members learn why food might taste the way it does, how food is transformed from the farm to the table, and discuss flavor, texture, and smell as constitutive parts of the experience of eating.

On a larger scale, Slow Food offers formal training in the education of taste. Their mission is to "promote and develop teaching activities on sensory education and food culture."[19] Slow Food offers a Master of Food degree where students study the origins, uses, and tastes of foods, the culture and history of gastronomy, and food science. More recently, however, the Slow Food movement has founded the Università di Scienze Gastronomiche, a university dedicated to "legitimizing the relationship between the field of gastronomy and the world of food production and agriculture."[20] The university "will supplement scientific learning with humanistic content and expand it with sensory and linguistic education (study of *terroirs* and artisans, of the history of the world's cuisines and foodstuffs and so on)."[21] At stake here is a broader notion of an epistemology of quality. Claims to knowledge are founded not only on a discourse of quantification, but must also account for geographic specificity, practical techniques, and taste—and thus must issue from a broader language employed by farmers, cooks, eaters, and scientists.

The kind of education offered by Slow Food is not restricted by a discourse of quantification, as is the case with the FDA and the USDA. Instead, a scientific discourse of quantification is a starting point for the development of a more subtle, complex, and well-developed epistemology. At the university, students are taught:

> How to choose raw materials, recognize products by taste, and document the history, geography and consumption of food. All these elements collectively make up a culture of knowledge and ideas that are essential for describing, producing, distributing, and selling food, and it is this culture that will be explored in depth at the University of Gastronomic Sciences. The University of Gastronomic Sciences will help to create a new type of professional: an expert who is able to lead and elevate the quality of production, to teach others how to taste, to guide the market, and to communicate about and promote foods and beverages. The University will provide those with an interest in understanding food with a humanistic, sensory approach, knowledge of traditional and industrial processes, and an appreciation of cooking and gastronomic tourism.[22]

In contrast to the well-educated eater constructed by the USDA, the person educated by Slow Food has both the intellectual and practical resources to talk about the science of nutrition, production and farming, and the experience and taste of specific foods.

Many convivia organize meetings around developing a sense of what particular foods taste like and subsequently learn about the production methods, cooking techniques, and nutritional portfolio of the foods. Taste is always considered just as important as science or farming at these events, and for Slow Food in general. For example, one required course in the Master of Food is Salamis and Cured Meats, which exhorts that "the sensory profile of salamis and cured meats deserves to be studied":[23]

> The first part of the course will seek to highlight the general quality of cured meats, while the second will be more specific, describing the distinctive characteristics of Italian regional varieties. The four lessons will cover everything from pig breeds and farms to production technologies and the use of salt and spices. Each lesson envisages guided tastings to evidence the principal sensory describers of boiled and raw salamis, lards and hams, as well as cured meats made from other animals, from geese to goats. The lessons will be attended by local producers.[24]

The master's degree treats food both scientifically and as an experience for the senses. For example, the cured meat course treats the science of food as a fundamental component but gives equal attention to the sensations and taste qualities as well. Learning to cure meat, and learning to appreciate the taste of cured meat, requires that the student understand the science behind meat curing, and the required ingredients, but this knowledge is not any more or less important than the ability to discern between and among sausages and develop personal preferences. The rhetorical purpose of Slow Food is to generate richer descriptions of experiences of eating—this is not a project of reduction but rather amplification.

Slow Food also publishes the periodical *Slow*, touting itself as the "international herald of tastes." This magazine contains articles that address a wide variety of foods, food producers, and global gastronomic affairs. But whether the issue is politics, growing techniques, or food science, a column called "Tasting Notes" is always included as a part of the process of understanding food. In the April 2003 issue, an extensive series of articles on beans describes where beans come from, bean farming techniques, the historic affiliation between beans and a culture of poverty, and most importantly tasting notes on eleven different kinds of beans. For example, the sweet flavor of the cuneo bean is "long-lasting with notes of chestnut," and the tolosa black bean "conjures up cinnamon and red wine" (p. 101). Thus, *Slow* creates its own discursive space for the development of a language of taste, and the effects of this new language are to augment and extend our available vocabulary for explaining taste.

In addition to *Slow*, the local convivia, and the university, Slow Food has established an Ark of Taste. The Ark aims to preserve "local gastronomic products threatened by industrial standardization, hyperhygienist legislation, the rules of the large-scale retail trade and the deterioration of the environment. The aim of the Ark of Taste is to rediscover, catalogue, describe and promote almost forgotten flavors."[25] Most importantly however, the Ark aims to unite gastronomic "experiences from around the world" and preserve foods that are "of exceptional quality, excellent in terms of taste and flavor."[26] The mission of Slow Food's Ark articulates the link between experience, taste, and food. In order for a food to be nominated to the Ark, a food must have cultural, geographic, or historical elements of experience that help describe the food's significance. In turn, these experiential factors help define a food's flavor, taste, and its "exceptional quality." As a metaphor the Ark acutely contrasts with the USDA's Food Pyramid with its focus on proportionality. No one flavor or experience is superior to another, and no flavor or taste can be organized by, or reduced to, its nutritional composition. Instead there are a plurality of flavors, experiences, and tastes, all worth preserving and celebrating.

The Slow Food movement demonstrates what is possible when a discourse of quantification is supplemented and extended by alternative languages. Not only does Slow Food offer an education in taste, but its publications, convivia, and general organization as a social movement all point to political, economic, and social agendas grounded on a discourse of taste. In contrast to the economic model of standardization established by the fast food industry, Slow Food advocates a "sustainable" approach to the economics of food. By grounding an economic model in tradition, geography, and taste, Slow Food articulates a radical critique of the capitalist reduction of food to a unit of exchange.[27] What is important is that the grounds of both a language that makes such a critique possible and the knowledge claims that give such a critique argumentative soundness cannot be reduced to a discourse of quantification. The complexity of food itself, as well as the complexity of the processes of farming, selling, and eating food, lends itself, from the perspective of Slow Food, to a plurality of languages that can account for the idiosyncrasy of experience while resisting the urge to standardization. Instead of focusing on profit, calories, or standard serving sizes, Slow Food makes possible an ongoing conversation about food that relies on community, flavor, taste, experience, tradition, land, and innumerable variables introduced by the members themselves and not mandated by any sole authority.

In many ways, this conversation is intended to oppose the effects of capitalism. During the 1980s and 1990s, both Slow Food and many food studies scholars were concerned with the rapid globalization of the food delivery system, most notably with the fast food industry (Leidner, 1993; Reiter, 1991; Ritzer, 1993; Watson, 1997). McDonald's has become an icon and universal symbol of American culture within this global food economy. And food magazines can be read not as vehicles for the preservation of the past but as forms of "food adventurism" (Heldke, 2003). Even discourses of soil or geography have been appropriated for political and economic ends (often free market, neoliberal ends). Free market rhetoric and consumer-oriented business practices can often undermine these claims to experience, or, worse, use such claims simply to increase efficiency and profit. In such cases, discourses of geography, history, and experience can be used to serve quantitative ends. Food studies scholarship has demonstrated the ways in which the food system has been bent to serve the interests of global capitalism and distort the rhetorical force of the alternative discourses I describe here (Watson and Caldwell, 2005). Such work is either indicative of the broader influence of quantification and the collaboration between nutrition science and global capitalism, or it can be read as a final attempt to subvert and control other kinds of claims that could authorize or legitimize our decisions about what to eat. Accordingly, Slow Food and the rise of farmers' markets can also be read as the last vestiges of resistance to the march of global capitalism and quantification. I prefer to read Slow Food, cookbooks, and websites like Chowhound in the latter fashion. Doing so, I believe, allows for the opportunity to cultivate a broader concept of public health located in authoritative discourses that extend beyond economics and science.

Beyond Quantification

A discourse of quantification can, and should, be supplemented with other languages whose various other goals offer a more complete picture of our relationship to food. Without accounting for other discursive practices and other communicative goals, federal nutrition policy will continue to fail because the language it employs fundamentally cannot achieve the communicative goals that other discourses achieve. As evidence of the fact that food and eating cannot be reduced to a discourse of quantification, I have pointed to several discursive spaces that intentionally supplement and transcend the language of science, that cannot be captured or reduced to numbers, and that avail themselves to multiple interpretations by grounding our notions of food more solidly on experiences of taste. The purpose of discourses that issue from taste, pleasure, flavor, experience, and tradition are to make communication about food a matter of conversation, disagreement, subjectivity, communality, localness, and the idiosyncratic. Such discourses provide a more complete picture of the complexity of food and eating and ground a larger variety of valid knowledge claims concerning notions of quality.

The discursive spaces that I have identified above are remarkable for their ability to unify people instead of dividing, classifying, and grouping people. Slow Food, for example, assumes that everyone has the discursive equipment to engage in conversations about flavor, taste, tradition, and geography, and encourages the sharing of experiences by different groups of people. Slow Food is designed to create local communities within which conversation is possible and knowledge about food is amplified to include the perspective of the farmer, the eater, and the cook. Within such communities, the process of communication is open-ended and lends itself to a multiplicity of competing and equally valid voices. The hope is that such communities will give rise to a deeper, richer, and more complete understanding of food. In contrast, a discourse of quantification has as its communicative goals the elimination of alternative voices, the silencing of the common perspective, and the domination of science over personal experience. Perhaps an ideally objective community could arise from a discourse of quantification, but such a community would lose all connection to the pursuit of pleasure, the familiarity of tradition, and the realm of possibility afforded by taste.

Within communities organized around discourses that privilege taste, the form of communication is also transformed. Instead of the transparency of an enumerated discourse, a discourse of experience employs words that have many interpretations. One hundred calories, as a description of a tablespoon of butter is a clear, concise, unwavering, and final statement. This sort of language does not encourage further conversation and has no other possible interpretations. Statements about the sweetness, the grassiness, or the sexiness of that butter issue from the experience of the eater, and encourage us to make claims about the quality of the butter. What is different is that such qualitative judgments are often founded on metaphor and encourage further descriptions, accounts, or explanations of the notion of good butter. In websites like chowhound.com, one can see the proliferation of such accounts, and one can also see how such a descriptive language effectively encourages this proliferation.

What is implied in the multiple threads on chowhound.com, the variety of available cookbooks, and the educational program advanced by Slow Food is the plurality of languages surrounding our relationship to food and the irreducibility of that plurality. The fundamental mistake of a discourse of quantification is its attempt to eliminate such plurality in favor of a single, unified voice. The irony is that as the food guides sought such a universal discourse of quantification, more and more numeric descriptors were invented, which caused greater confusion. Discourses that privilege taste encourage the development of many languages, and gain descriptive strength, communicative dexterity, and evaluative purchase from manyness. Being able to describe both food and eating from a multiplicity of perspectives and with a multiplicity of languages allows one access to aspects of food that are inaccessible using a discourse of quantification.

Discourses that issue from history, geography, and experience use themes like home, tradition, seasonality, locality, conversation, conviviality, and pleasure to establish valid mechanisms for knowing quality without relying on measurements, standards, and repeatability tests. The examples of these discourses that I have chosen provide new discursive tools with which one may reconstruct our conceptions of nutrition and health. The purpose of engaging in discourses of history, geography, and experience is to provide one with the ability to evaluate a discourse of quantification, identifying its shortcomings and its benefits. It is also to establish grounds upon which alternative epistemologies are and have been founded, and to draw a discourse of quantification into conversation with different discourses. The hope is that this conversation will create a fuller understanding of food, taste, and the act of eating. The sources identified here are only the beginning for such a task. The trouble lies in the dominance of a discourse of quantification and its insistence on discounting the viability of the more accessible and more subjective alternatives.

Conclusion

Rethinking Common Sense

Toward a Rhetoric of Eating

Pushing my cart through the grocery aisles recently, I came upon something, or was it nothing? I wasn't sure. Next to the bags of prewashed greens (a good source of folic acid and vitamin C) stood a display of salad dressing. It was salad dressing of the white, creamy sort. "Calorie Free, Fat Free, No Carbs!" the label proclaimed. The only nutritional component the label had left out was protein, but knowing that the dressing contained "no calories" meant that that was absent as well. I was looking at the equivalent of the gastronomic simulacrum. It looked like something was there, but nothing was. Nutritionally and figuratively, this was a bottle of nothing. I looked at the label more closely and began reading the nutrition facts. This product contributed 0% of the daily calories of a 2,000-calorie-per-day-diet, and none of the recommended calcium, carbohydrates, or protein. Scanning the numbers, I noticed that it *did* contain sodium, but I suppose that wasn't considered a salient point, since the USDA urges us to reduce our sodium. To the rational thinker this would seem absurd. Why would anyone pay $3.99 to put *nothing* on a salad, and, why would a company use a discourse of quantification to advertise that they are selling nothing? "Nothing" came in 15 flavors including French, Country Italian, Russian, Bacon Ranch, and Bleu Cheese, and, I suppose, this product sought to convince shoppers to buy one of these flavors simply on the grounds that they could eat without consuming anything.

The existence of this salad dressing illustrates my concern that a food's quantities have become its qualities, and that those quantities (whether it is portion size, RDAs, calories, or fat content) are used as a basis for judging the quality of a food. In this case the salad dressing's quantities—which were, in essence, the quantification of things that weren't there—were its selling points, the things that made it "good," appealing, and presumably marketable. Numbers, measurements, and statistics have become gastronomic markers, or replacements for quality, taste, and tradition. This project has illustrated the history of this quantitative language and how that language became the default manner of communication about food. I have shown where this discourse was first applied to food, and how it proliferated under the auspices of the U.S. Department of Agriculture. Underlying this flourishing discourse was a historical context of progress, order, and standardization. This context created an environment in which science was a social ideal, a progressive, helpful theme, as well as a discursive framework. Numbers, in this context, form the basis for rationales and epistemologies that are methodical, rigorous, and special in that they are "created" by experts.

Using USDA publications as resources, I have shown that the messages of each food guide were timely and situational. Politics, economics, and social structure dictated the content of an individual food guide's message: strength during wartime, parsimony during economic hardship, and health during economic booms. But as the content of each food guide changed, the form was unwavering. From the first guide published in 1917, numbers defined food, standards defined eaters, and measuring replaced eating. The food guides abstracted eating from tradition, history, and location. One did not eat because he or she enjoyed food; one ate to attain standards, to gain health through various nutrients, and to reach numeric goals so that he or she might consider himself or herself a complete eater. Certain foods were "good" or "bad" based on their numbers and their ability to help the eater achieve nutritional goals. Quality food met scientific standards, and one was encouraged to judge food on these criteria. A discourse of quantification allowed the USDA to normalize Americans based on what they needed to eat.

Therefore, I have shown how intertwined and reliant discussions of food and nutrition have become upon a discourse of quantification. In chapter 3, I claimed that even in the face of a new nutritional problem—Americans were eating too much food instead of too little—the government's approach to defining and solving this problem consisted of simply redefining qualitative terms like good and bad with new quantities. Thus, even though "good" shifted to "less" and "bad" shifted to "more," in discussions of calories, fat, sodium, and cholesterol, the USDA remained committed to a quantitative understanding of food. In addition to official diet recommendations, alternative solutions to America's nutrition problems were trapped in a discourse of quantification as well. Those giving nutritional advice that differed from the USDA's message, like Walter Willett, employed a discourse of quantification to make their criticisms. These critics underscore this project's main argument. In order to legitimately critique the food guides and recommend alternative nutrition plans, one had to use the language of science. Critics who claimed to have "alternatives" to the USDA guidelines may have been alternative in the content of their message, but not in the form.

This history, then, is a history of the official rhetoric of food and eating that was invented, disseminated, and managed by the collusion between science and the U.S. government beginning in the late 19th century. This rhetoric has formed the "common sense" view of food and eating in America. The most powerful and persuasive effect of the discourse of quantification has been its ability to produce the belief that science and quantification can tell us all that we need to know about food and eating. The French Paradox is an excellent illustration of this effect. The health benefits of wine could only be understood through, and reduced to, a kind of scientific common sense. We have come to assume that calories are the essential, constitutive component of the foods that we eat, and that by regulating our caloric intake we will have healthy, fully functioning bodies. We assume that the Nutrition Facts labels pasted onto the packages of foods we buy are an unequivocally good by-product of government and science working in the interests of the public. More and more, cultural practices are matters of counting, comparing, and explaining. This book has sought to show that this common sense has a history, and is, itself, not the inevitable progress of science but a product of social organization, political decision-making, and communicative practices.

To use a term from the history of rhetoric, most cultural objects or practices have a *doxa*. *Doxa* refers to views that are self-evident, common, social, or cultural beliefs. It is often thought of in relationship to *episteme* or true, systemic knowledge. The problem with the history of nutrition is that it presents scientific advice about diet and health as an *episteme*, and assumes that this *episteme* should form the basis for our common sense. But American beliefs about food vary greatly from the beliefs of other cultures. The French Paradox is an example of incommensurable *doxa*. The French have their own common sense view of the place of food in their culture, and it has nothing to do with calories, proteins, or serving sizes. French cultural practices contribute to a *doxastic* view of health that is also part of a larger body of social knowledge, and drinking wine is part of that conception of health. American hubris has led to the position that all other *doxa* can be explained by a scientific *episteme* of nutrition. This is a uniquely American kind of common sense. From the perspective of the rhetorical tradition, we have confused *doxa* and *episteme*. Nutrition is not an *episteme*; it has become a uniquely American *doxa*. In other words, nutrition is best viewed as a way of understanding food and eating in terms of quantities and scientific explanations; it is not a closed system of true knowledge. By virtue of scientists like Wilbur Atwater, symbols like the Food Pyramid, and population studies about serving sizes, we have come to believe that food and eating can and should be reduced to numbers and scientific explanations. But food and eating, as I contend in chapter 5, cannot be reduced to, defined by, or explained solely in terms of science and quantification.

My intention in this book is to tell a critical history. The purpose of a critical history is to rethink the common sense view that now holds such persuasive power in our culture. In other words, it is to question whether or not the current *doxa* represents beliefs worth holding to. Therefore, one must test the effects of the *doxastic* beliefs that inform food and eating in America. But, and the USDA is well aware of this, it is clear, by all accounts, that government-sanctioned dietary advice has been a massive failure. This is the cause of the paradox I referred to in the introduction: there is a concomitant rise in diseases related to diet *and* an increasing body of sound, scientific knowledge regarding the link between diet and health. Clearly, a discourse of quantification, as a communicative strategy, is an unquestionable failure. In other words, communication by quantification has not been able to link scientific, dietary advice with actual eating practices. Perhaps this is because when people eat they do not eat like scientists performing experiments in the lab. In any case, clearly the problem does not lie with the knowledge that has been produced but with the strategies used for public communication. A discourse of quantification cannot, and does not, achieve the desired goals of improved public health—it only quantifies health. For this reason, we must challenge the view that foods are best reduced to calories and that eating is a matter of matching energy output with caloric input. This kind of common sense has not produced healthy bodies. One could argue, and perhaps this is for another book written at another time, that a discourse of quantification has, in fact, contributed to the growing incidence of diet-related disease by destroying other forms of common sense that were better at producing and sustaining health, but that argument is beyond the scope of this project.

According to my critical history, then, the official rhetoric of food and eating that has emerged over the last hundred years or so is incomplete, ineffective, and inadequate. Our common sense view of food and eating does not represent a right and true representation of what food really is, but instead tropes food, certifies a quantitative reality, and attempts to eradicate other knowledge claims based on history, geography, experience, and tradition. The science of nutrition has refigured food, in the name of public health, and in so doing, has manufactured a way of knowing and judging our relationships to food and health that is abstract, numeric, and overly functional. An alternative rhetoric of eating would require a broader vocabulary, a different way of figuring food, and a new system of knowing and judging what to eat. Only by refiguring food, eating, and health in other ways can we hope to solve the paradox of increasing rates of diet-related diseases alongside increasing scientific evidence about the relationship between diet and health. In other words, we need a new language that describes food and eating in such a way that communicative practices are actually capable of producing public health. This does not mean disregarding or ignoring the last hundred years of nutrition research and scientific evidence. Nor does it mean eliminating the use of numbers in discussions of food. But it does mean attempting to understand food, eating, and health in ways that are not simply reduced to mathematical formulae.

This is an enormously difficult task. New languages, new discourses, and new versions of common sense do not develop over night. Often that kind of work is a product of institutional change, large-scale social reorganization, and the recreation or redescription of broad and complex notions like "health" (all of which can be glacial at best). In other words, one book does not make a revolution. To dislodge the common sense approach to food that has taken over 100 years to solidify itself is tantamount to claiming that we need to remake American culture from the ground up—from that perspective, the task seems impossible. The good news, however, is that such change does happen. In the 19th century, to understand diet in terms of calories and portions was unthinkable. My hope is that by the end of the 21st century a new kind of common sense will have emerged that is unthinkable from our perspective. But such a process must start with a challenge to the status quo and I hope that this book is taken as one such challenge.

This book, then, seeks a rhetoric of food and eating that extends beyond the common sense view provided by nutrition research. Moreover, I insist that a rhetoric of eating must extend beyond a discourse of quantification if we are to promote and qualitatively improve public health. This is another way of saying that such a rhetoric is necessary given the failures of the current rhetoric to accomplish the goals that it has set for itself. Such a rhetoric would not be reductionist and would not eliminate the importance of culture, tradition, geography, and experience, but would celebrate and affirm such concepts as having a vital place in the construction of a new American *doxa*. Such a rhetoric would not treat all American eaters as ethically incomplete or functionally the same, but would learn to build from the existing, idiosyncratic cultural traditions that we already have in order to certify eating practices that celebrate taste as an important feature of health. It would treat food as more than fuel and eating as more than a function, and thus would have the possibility of actually communicating the advances of science in a way that would make public understanding possible. Persuasion begins with establishing a common ground between audience members (Perelman and Olbrechts-Tyteca, 1969). The USDA never took this step, and that is why its techniques continue to miss the mark. This is to suggest that if the USDA wants the public to heed nutritional advice, such advice must come in a language that accounts for the culture and experience of their audience. I do not wish to discount science or nutrition, but I do wish to show how that knowledge can be supplemented with alternative discourses to more effective ends.

Over the course of this book, I have explored the discursive inter-action between science and food in the U.S. Department of Agriculture, its administrators, and its publications. I have shown how a discourse of quantification was conceived, how it was routinely applied by the USDA, and how it works to persuade. I have also offered an alternative set of discourses to supplement a discourse of quantification. These discourses are plural and subjective in nature. They contrast with the objectivity and univocality of a discourse of quantification. The discourse of quan-tification is useful and helpful—but it cannot be the only language we use to communicate ideas about the food we eat. Eating is a sensory experience—to abstract food by calculation denies us certain qualities of experience. My hope is to reclaim food with these alternative discourses so that our understanding and determination of "good" food takes place on and within the palates and farms and memories of all people, and not a select scientific community. I am not calling for the abandonment of a discourse of quantification, only that we place this discourse on the plate with other discursive options.

Understanding a discourse of quantification and its tropes, and being able to identify the types of arguments that underpin a discourse of quantification, creates a context for the development of a supplemen-tal language. This language, which draws its authority from subjective experiences like taste, history, or geography, can balance a discourse of quantification by giving eaters an opportunity to create their own set of criteria for determining "quality" food—criteria that require hunger, experience, community, and family traditions. This begs many questions: Would the USDA be better off attempting to speak to the public using the themes of chapter 5? Instead of publishing a Food Pyramid, should the USDA simply tell people to eat whatever, whenever, and however? Instead of encouraging the public to know their quantitative "good" and "bad" fats, would a better approach be to encourage the eater to judge food solely on its taste? Instead of rating the quality of food on its nutritional portfolio, should we rate quality food on where it is from or how it makes us feel? The answer to these questions is both yes and no.

Any rhetoric of food and eating is incomplete and inadequate if it does not take culture, geography, tradition, experience, and taste into consideration along with the nutritional composition of foods and health. I would not go so far as to suggest that any rhetoric could be complete, in the sense that it could describe and explain all that we needed to know about food and eating. But I would argue that some rhetorics are fuller, richer, more complex, and better able to understand and explain the role of food in producing health and culture than some other rhetorics. In this case, the official rhetoric of the USDA is an impoverished one, and it is for that reason that the USDA continues to fail in improving public health. This is not to say that the science of nutrition is not helpful or important for such tasks, but it is to suggest that when communicative practices are limited and highly technical, in the manner that I have shown them to be in official U.S. dietary advice, they do not, and cannot, achieve all that they seek to achieve.

Quantitative discourse, numeric organization, science, and objectivity are important features of large and complex public health issues. At one level, creating and giving the public a certain kind of knowledge, and fostering a particular discourse that facilitates the normalization of the population is not a bad thing. For example, in discussions of public health it behooves the USDA to have a concrete and transparent language with which they can determine who needs federal resources, where these needs reside, and how to get those resources to the needy. A discourse of quantification is useful because it can provide information about public health trends. Looking at a current nutritional map of the United States, it is clear that obesity is a major problem. According to the Centers for Disease Control, in the year 2002, 20 states had obesity prevalence rates of 15–19%; 29 states had rates of 20–24%; and 1 state reported a rate over 25 percent. Ten years prior, only four states had an obesity prevalence rate of 15–19%, and none had a rate above 20%. It is quite possible that quantification is responsible for the trend of recognizing obesity as a health crisis rather than, to take one example, a manifestation of human diversity.

Regardless, this information is taken to be shocking and disturbing, but this is largely because we can use the discourse of quantification to invent and enumerate the problem and subsequently compare numeric data sets. This particular affliction has a host of corollary health problems that lower life expectancy and raise healthcare costs and risk factors for other maladies like depression, heart disease, and stroke. Without a quantitative discursive system in place to determine both how severe the problem is (using Body Mass Indices, Activity Levels, Caloric Intake, etc.) and methods for abating that problem (Maximizing Calories Burned During Exercise, Metabolism Studies, Elimination of Partially Hydrogenated Fats, etc.), the problem appears insurmountable. If people eat, or ate, according to the USDA food guides, they would achieve the goals that each food guide purports to have. For example, if you learned the difference between an enumerated "good" and "bad" fat, you *would* be on the way to a "healthier" diet. But this version of health is strictly quantitative. In other words, the obesity statistics demonstrate the erosion of qualitative conceptions of health. It is almost surely the case that qualitative conceptions of health would frame obesity differently.

In all of the cases I have studied here, there are numerically defined problems and numerically defined solutions, and by articulating the problems with numbers, we hope to be able to predict the outcome, but we cannot. It is at this point that a discourse of quantification demonstrates its inability to completely define and address the issue of what constitutes good American food. Enumerated discussions of food, and quantified notions of the American eater, work very well when used as models to predict our problems and solutions and as theories to explain those problems and solutions. A discourse of quantification is appealing and persuasive because it has no contingency. It defines situations in no uncertain terms, and that surety is comforting, solid, and reliable. An osteoporotic woman who drinks a glass of milk at every meal can be sure that she is taking in 1,000 milligrams of calcium. She has likely been told that milk is a "good" source of calcium. Her like or dislike for milk, her preference for collard greens, or her backyard fig tree (both which are "good" sources of calcium as well) are irrelevant. Her numerically defined condition, and the numerically prescribed solution are well matched.

The problem for a discourse of quantification arises when the "eater" becomes a real individual—someone with taste buds, a memory, a community, and personal relationships. At every meal, each person brings with them a body of knowledge about food. Some of this knowledge is quantitative, but much of it is historical, geographic, and experiential. This qualitative knowledge arises from myriad discourses of taste and grows with every eating experience. Each time we try a new food and discover we like it, or we convene at a family dinner, or we eat something we have grown or raised ourselves, we build upon these discourses of taste. The frequency of these situations forces us to find new ways to express "good" food, to describe taste, and to recollect eating experiences. It is this mutability, and situational adaptability, that a discourse of quantification lacks. We cannot measure the sweet taste of the first bite of wedding cake of a newly married couple. We can only measure how many calories are in the buttercream icing. We cannot count why the first ripe peach of summer tastes the best, we can only know how many grams of fiber it has. We cannot quantify why two spanakopitas from two next-door neighbors mean different things to the two families that eat them. We can only know that one serving of spanakopita represents one serving of vegetables, and equals one-third of the daily allowance of saturated fat. The discourses that I address in chapter 5 all attempt to capture these intangible and unquantifiable aspects of food and eating. They are attempts at describing the ephemeral quality and subjectivity of eating. And they are modes of talk that recognize the individuality of taste and celebrate a plurality of voices, without attempting to override those voices with a singular objective voice. While a discourse of quantification attempts to control, discourses of taste acknowledge the contingency of individuals, and how and what they eat. To match these two inclinations would be to move beyond the common sense view of food and eating that we have inherited from the science of nutrition, and to move toward an improved rhetoric.

Notes

Chapter 1. The Early History of American Nutrition Research

1. Prior to the formation of the USDA, all agricultural issues were handled by the Patent Office. The first commissioner of the USDA, a former Pennsylvanian farmer named Isaac Newton, was the previous chief of the agricultural section of the Patent Office. In that same year, 1862, the U.S. Congress passed the Homestead Act that allowed any American citizen, or any alien who intended to become a citizen, 160 acres of land in the American West, for a $10 registration fee. Almost half a million people applied for homesteads, but because the land in the West was so dry, it was difficult for the homesteaders to make an agricultural living from the land. One reason that the establishment of the Department of Agriculture was concurrent with the Homestead Act was that this may have been a way for the government to research ways to maximize agricultural productivity on arid land.

2. United States Congress. Senate, 37th Congress, 2nd Session. An Act to Establish a Department of Agriculture, May 15, 1862, Chapter 72, Bill 249.

3. Work to ensure food purity began in the USDA in the Division of Chemistry in 1883 with the examination and comparison of regional domestic butters. Among the adulterants were: tallow, lard, oleomargarine, and cottonseed oil. Food adulteration, as well as public health issues, and labor violations were addressed in Upton Sinclair's *The Jungle*, a novel exposing the deplorable conditions of the meatpacking industry in Chicago. This text, along with the work of USDA chemist Dr. Harvey W. Wiley, is rumored to have been the impetus behind the passage of the Pure Food and Drug Act in 1906.

4. It should be noted that while the Morrill Land Grant College Act and the establishment of the USDA occurred during the Civil War, neither measure used the war as a rationale for their passage or formation. In *Agriculture and the Civil War*, Paul Gates (1965) argues that the Morrill Act was "one of the important measures enacted by the Federal government during the Civil War" because it reaffirmed the government's commitment to education and maintained its deep roots "in the American way of life" (p. 251). Between 1862 and 1865, the Morrill Act applied only to the North. After 1865 the measure was extended

179

to the South, thus states both above and below the Mason-Dixon line would have resources with which they could develop their own agricultural research. At the time the USDA was formed, farming was "full of vitality . . . and revealed a remarkable amount of variety" (Gates, 1965, p. vii), and it was expanding rapidly to the Northwest and Southwest.

5. U.S. Department of Agriculture, Remarks of M. H. Buckam, Proceedings of the Thirteenth Annual Convention of the Association of American Agricultural Colleges and Experiment Stations, Held at San Francisco, CA, July 5–6, 1899, *Office of Experiment Stations Bulletin* no. 76 (Washington, DC: Government Printing Office, 1900), p. 34.

6. In *No Other Gods*, Charles Rosenberg (1976) argues that economics and the goal of financially profitable American farms frequently goaded the experiment stations' work. The rationalization and systematization that scientific study could bring to agriculture would, in theory, help to increase production yields and would "help the farmers adjust to an increasingly competitive world market" (p. 154). Many apolitical and unaffiliated advocates of the experiment stations lauded them as being a true and earnest boon to American farmers, performing time-consuming, systematic research that the average farmer could not possibly do.

7. A eudiometer is an apparatus for measuring the change in the volume of gases during a chemical reaction.

8. The consolidation of Liebig's approach to nutrition was certainly not inevitable. Jacob Moleschott had a distinctly different, humanistic perspective on nutrition during that same period (see Kamminga and Cunningham, 1995, pp. 15–47). However, several factors including Liebig's success at training chemists in his lab helped solidify his particular perspective on nutrition as the only viable perspective.

9. See Wilbur O. Atwater, U.S. Department of Agriculture, "Agricultural-Experiment Stations in Europe" Report of the Commissioner of Agriculture for the Year 1875. (Washington, DC: Government Printing Office, 1876), pp. 517–524.

10. Hatch Act 1887, Sec. 1–2, Chapter 314, 49th Congress, Session 2, March 2, 1887.

11. The USDA nutrition cause had an ally in wealthy Massachusetts business-man Edward Atkinson, who believed that American capitalism was in crisis and looked to cheaper and more nutritious food as a solution to this crisis. Around the time that the Hatch Act was to be passed, Atkinson published a series of articles in *Century* magazine discussing and comparing national and international food habits and the subsequent "strength" of the nations. See Edward Atkinson, "The Food Question in America and Europe," *Century* 33 (1886–1887): 238–248; "The Relative Strength and Weakness of Nations," *Century* 33 (1886–1887): 423–435 and 613–621; and "The Margins of Profits," *Century* 33 (1886–1887): 923–931.

12. Hatch Act 1887, Sec. 3, Chapter 314, 49th Congress, Session 2, March 2, 1887.

13. U.S. Department of Agriculture, Report of the Director of the Office of Experiment Stations for 1889 (Washington, DC: Government Printing Office, 1889); and U.S. Department of Agriculture Report of the Director of the

Office of Experiment Stations for 1890 (Washington, DC: Government Printing Office, 1890).

14. Both Rubner's and Voit's ideas of the human machine had, according to Cravens, "large ideological import." Concurrent with the hard science approach to the human body by scientists like Rubner and Voit, there was an opposing view expounded by the vitalists. The vitalists maintained that the living and nonliving forms of nature had qualitative differences. By arguing that the human body worked according to the same principles as a steam engine, the chemical nutritionists successfully challenged the theologians, clerics, poets, and philosophers ideas regarding life and nature.

15. Rubner's calorimetric experimentation served as the foundation for isodynamic law, where he established that 100 grams of fat was equivalent to 211 grams of protein, and roughly 240 grams of starch or sugar. These findings led to the Rubner factors of "calories per gram" for protein, fats, and carbohydrates: 4.1, 9.3, and 4.1 respectively. While these numbers were very similar to Atwater's later discovery of the 4, 9, and 4 calories/gram of protein, fats and carbohydrates, Rubner's data did not consider how digestion may affect the caloric energy available in certain foods. Thus Atwater, who did extensive work on the digestibility of foods in conjunction with calorimetry, is credited with the discovery. See Buford Nichols's "Atwater and USDA Nutrition Research and Service: A Prologue of the Past Century," *The Journal of Nutrition* 124 (1994): 1724S–1725S.

16. Between the years 1875 and 1881 Atwater published 69 articles in *American Agriculturalist* entitled "Science Applied to Farming" that encouraged the application of scientific knowledge to practical farming. He also published, in 1894 in the *Farmers' Bulletin* no. 23, an article entitled "Foods, Nutritive Value and Cost," which was aimed at housewives and served as perhaps the first federally issued food guide.

17. This amount increased to $15,000 in the fiscal year of 1897.

18. Atwater's figures of 4, 9, and 4 calories per gram of digestible protein, fats, and carbohydrates have not been challenged since his late 19th-century studies. Twentieth-century calorimetry tests at the USDA center for nutrition in Beltsville, MD, have determined that Atwater's units are correct.

19. After Atwater pioneered domestic respiration calorimetry, other experiment stations began to adapt the apparatus to farm animals to determine the available energy of various types of fodder. Experiments were first done with steer and timothy hay where it was determined that for cattle the caloric equation depended on tissue replacement rather than heat production. Besides large numbers of analyses of animal feed, the USDA studied the composition of beef, mutton, pork, and poultry fattened and fed in different conditions.

20. Atwater saw nutrition primarily in terms of its ability to improve the physical strength of laboring men. Because men were the wage earners, they were most in need of nutritious foods, and to consider them the prototype for his studies that determined "nutritional requirements per pound of body weight" was safe, and even generous to the nutritional needs of women and children, whose levels of activity would be considerably less. See Atwater's "Food and Diet" (1895) in the *1894 Yearbook of Agriculture*.

21. By 1907 experiment stations performed more than 100 studies and published 56 different "dietaries" of a variety of cultures, races, ages, and professions.

Chapter 2. Reading Federal Nutrition Guides

1. The USDA published the first food guide in 1916, which was aimed at teaching mothers how to feed their children. I have chosen to begin with the first food guide aimed at the adult public.

2. The use of the word "common" is ironic considering the fact that the USDA defined the family, the foods and parameters under which one should eat. "Commonly used foods" could be anything that the USDA wanted them to be, just as the definition of the "American home" was up to their discretion as well.

3. In the 1933 guide, Stiebeling attempts to clear up the grading system. In her discussion of fruits and vegetables, Stiebeling is quick to point out that just because a food is labeled B or C grade does not mean that the quality of the food is bad. It means that the substandard food may not be "up to the recognized standard in some other respect" and that "products which carry the substandard labeling are wholesome food" (41).

4. The discovery of vitamin B₁ by Casimir Funk in 1912 was the first recognition of the link between certain substances and the incidence of disease. Funk noticed that an increase in the intake of polished rice (rice that lacked the outer grain) was concurrent with the incidence of beriberi. Funk surmised that there was something in the grain that had the power to prevent disease and called the substance a "vitamine" by combining the words "vital" and "amine." He called the substance a "vitamine" because he had isolated a nitrogenous substance from the polishings of the rice. While Funk is credited with discovering vitamins, in 1906 Sir Frederick Hopkins made note of an "accessory food factor," some essential component of food. It was Funk, however, who established the link between food and disease.

5. War Food Administration. *Proceedings of the National Nutrition Conference for Defense*, May 26–28, 1941 (Washington, DC: Government Printing Office, 1942), p. viii.

6. At the time, the important vitamins and minerals that the chart recommended were: calcium, iron, vitamin A, thiamin (vitamin B₁), riboflavin, nicotinic acid (now known as niacin), ascorbic acid (vitamin C), and vitamin D. The units for measure were a combination of grams, milligrams, and IU (international units), an obscure measurement that, unless one was familiar with laboratory practice, or had access to a precise scientific measuring apparatus, would not be common. In addition to these microscopic measurements, the chart also specified daily calorie and protein intake.

7. War Food Administration, *Proceedings of the National Nutrition Conference for Defense*, May 26–28, 1941, p. v.

8. When the RDAs were published and presented at the May 1941 Committee of Food and Nutrition meeting, they bore the title *Yardstick for Good*

Nutrition. The push for Americans to compare themselves to sets of numbers was even represented in the title and iconography of a ruler pictured on the cover.

9. USDA, *National Wartime Food Guide* (Washington, DC: Government Printing Office, Rev. July, 1943).

10. Office of War Information, *Food Rationing and the War—An Address by Mr. Elmer Davis,* December 27, 1942 (Washington, DC: Government Printing Office, 1942).

11. This suggestion by the USDA that Americans now had access to more food and more types of food is a misnomer. Many Americans saw their diet improve during the war because rations made certain quantities of certain foods available to the public, when before they were difficult to come by.

Chapter 3. The Food Pyramid

1. U.S. Department of Agriculture, *USDA's Food Guide: Background and Development,* Human Nutrition Information Service Miscellaneous Publication No. 1514 (Washington, DC: Government Printing Office, September 1993), p. 19.

2. As early as the 1960s the Red Cross and the American Heart Foundation had published guides to lowering sodium intake and the perils of being overweight. The USDA published *Food and Your Weight* in 1968 and revised it in 1973 as well as *Calories and Weight* in 1981. The "Hunger in America" documentary broadcast on May 21, 1968, used hunger as the guise for reporting on poverty in America. All of the "malnutrition" cases the documentary covered were the urban and rural poor.

3. U.S. Department of Agriculture, *Legislative History of the Select Committee on Nutrition and Human Needs* (Washington, DC: Government Printing Office, 1976), pp. 40–41.

4. Senate Resolution 281 Report No. 1416, July 30, 1968, 90th Congress, 2nd Session.

5. U.S. Department of Agriculture, *Hearings before the Select Committee on Nutrition and Human Needs and the United States Senate, Part One: Problems and Prospects* (Washington, DC: Government Printing Office, 1969), pp. 7–8.

6. The committee consisted of seven senators and one chairman. While the USDA demonstrated their faith in science, three of the senators on the committee gave a supplement to the report that stated their skepticism about the link between intake of animal fat and disease and urged that the goals state in bold print "the value of dietary change remains controversial and science cannot at this time insure that an altered diet will provide improved protection from certain killer diseases such as heart disease and cancer."

7. U.S. Department of Agriculture, *Hearings of the 64th Select Committee on Nutrition and Human Needs of the U.S. Senate, 95th Congress, 1st Session, Part 1 Cardiovascular Disease,* February 1–2, 1977 (Washington, DC: Government Printing Office, 1977), p. 289. On March 24, 1977, Bob Dole, then a Kansas senator, mollified the president of the National Cattleman's Association by proposing the amendment of dietary goal number 2 from "decrease consumption of

meat" to "increase consumption of lean meat," to which the president replied "decrease is a bad word senator."

8. It is interesting to note that the salt and cholesterol intake limits were set in metric grams, units familiar to scientists only.

9. This continued role of the USDA in nutrition policy came in 1977 with Congress granting the Department of Health, Education and Welfare (DHEW, the precursor to the DHHS) and the Department of Agriculture joint responsibility for a range of nutrition activities including distributing dietary advice to the public. The Farm Bill (Public Law 95–113) that united the two departments was crafted in part due to the lack of "prevention" initiative of the DHEW.

10. In the supplemental foreword of the December 1977 version of the dietary goals, Senators Percy, Schweiker, and Zorinsky voiced their disdain for the dietary goals' lack of conclusive scientific evidence. They cited "an impressive lack of agreement among scientists on the efficacy of dietary change" and noted that "it is clear that science has not progressed to the point where we can recommend to the general public that cholesterol intake be limited to a specific amount. . . . A similar divergence of scientific opinion on the question of whether dietary change can help the heart illustrates that science can not yet verify with any certainty that coronary heart disease will be prevented or delayed by the diet recommended in this report."

11. Marion Nestle (2002) describes the machinations of the selection of the food pyramid over the bowl design (p. 63). Bell Associates determined that neither the bowl nor the pyramid were particularly effective in communicating the information to the children and low-income focus groups, but because so much time and money had been invested in the project, the time had come for the USDA to release the food guide. Nestle indicates that the USDA was faced with a dilemma. Selecting the pyramid over the bowl would make the USDA's extra research and tax dollars spent redundant, since the pyramid was ready for release nearly a year earlier, and selecting the bowl would make the USDA seem subservient to industry pressure.

Chapter 4. Scaling the Pyramid

1. After the controversy surrounding industry influence on nutritional guidance had died down, the USDA orchestrated a new release of its Food Guide Pyramid. Many of the newspaper columnists who had been very critical of the USDA during its "waffling" period between May 1991 and May 1992 remained fairly critical after the Pyramid's release.

2. By the mid to late 1990s several publications used the word "epidemic" in describing the rapid spread of obesity. The *Journal of the American Medical Association* (October 27, 1999) published a study that showed that between the years of 1991 and 1998, the prevalence of obesity had increased in every state of the union by anywhere from 11% in Delaware to 101% in Georgia. By 1998, at least 22% of the American population was obese, that is to say 30 pounds or more overweight. Dr. David Satcher, then U.S. surgeon general, published a "Call to Action to Prevent and Decrease Overweight and Obesity" in 2001 that highlighted

the "surfacing of an epidemic." In January of 2000 Marion Nestle and Michael Jacobson of the New York University Department of Nutrition and Food Studies and the Center for Science in the Public Interest coauthored an article in *Public Health Reports* entitled "Halting the Obesity Epidemic: A Public Health Policy Approach" that made several policy recommendations to deal with the problem.

3. It is interesting to note that the USDA attempted to address "culture" by creating links on their website to alternative "Ethnic/Cultural" Pyramids. For example, the Asian Food Pyramid places noodles, rice, and rice products at the bottom of the Pyramid. The alcoholic beverage to be consumed in moderation is sake. Other pyramids include the Native American Food Pyramid (which looks strikingly similar to the USDA Pyramid) and the Vegetarian Pyramid, whose meat group consists largely of soy-based products, nuts and nut butters, and eggs. Oldways also uses "traditional" cultures to create food pyramids. Their Latin American Food Pyramid suggests servings of cherimoya and guanabana in the fruit group; malanga, taro, and arepas in the starch group; and tomatillos and cactus in their vegetable group.

4. On September 11, 2003, the USDA called for key revisions to the Food Guide Pyramid, one of which stated the new food guide will start "using 'cups' and 'ounces' vs. 'servings' in consumer materials to suggest daily amounts to choose from each food group and subgroup" (USDA, 2003).

5. In the actual food guide publication, the meat and milk industry pressure that caused such controversy in the preempted 1991 release of the Pyramid becomes ever more clear. While the meat industry lost the battle for a different visual icon to make meats seem equally as important as the grains, fruits, and vegetables, the Food Pyramid actually increased the recommended intake of meat from 4–6 ounces in the Basic Four guide to 5–7 ounces in the Food Guide Pyramid. The Basic Four recommended 2 servings per day. The *Dietary Guidelines for Americans* that are released every five years have increased their recommendation from 6 ounces of meat per day in 1990 to an upper limit to 9 ounces per day in the 5th edition of the guidelines published in 2000.

6. In "A Little 'Lite' Reading," the FDA introduced new federally quantified regulations that dictated what words food manufacturers could use to describe the qualities of their package contents. There were 11 core terms that the FDA defined: free, low, lean, extra-lean, high, good source, reduced, less, light, fewer, and more. For example, "light" or "lite" meant that the package contained "a nutritionally altered product that contained one-third fewer calories or half the fat of the reference food. If the food derives 50 percent or more of its calories from fat, the reduction must be 50 percent of the fat." Just as with the term "serving," the government imbued these terms with quantitative meaning. But these terms also implied health benefits when referenced with the Food Guide Pyramid. Because the Food Guide Pyramid disparaged fat, fat-free is a desirable quality of a food, as is extra-lean. Presumably, "a good source of fat" printed on the label would make consumers leery of the food, just as "reduced vitamins" or "nutrient-lite." This regulation of the 11 core terms certified the quantitative nature of foods and provided an epistemological language for food talk.

7. Food and Drug Administration Publication, 21 CFR Part 101, "Food Labeling: Nutrient Content Claims, General Principles; Health Claims, General

Requirements and Other Specific Requirements for Individual Health Claims."
Docket 94P-0390, p. 66208.

8. The food survey data, based on the report "Continuing Survey of Food
Intakes by Individuals" (CSFII 1989–1991) indicates that in most cases all ages
of men and women ate more than one serving per eating occasion, and, in many
cases, the typical amount eaten at each sitting was equal to 2 or 3 times the
government-determined serving.

9. Attempts to quantify tradition and custom result in the clash of the
subjective and the objective on every occasion. An Orthodox Jew when asked
how much pork they customarily eat at every occasion would necessarily answer
"none." But this number would obscure the actual factors that regulate eating
practices. It is not because of diet that the Orthodox Jew rejects pork, but rather
because of tradition, religion, and culture.

10. The American media also had a fascination with comparing the American
portions and servings with the "cuisine minceur" of France (Callahan, 2003). The
average size of the French portion of ice cream, for example, is a golf ball, while
an American average serving size of an ice cream scoop is a tennis ball.

11. Marion Nestle (2002) describes the strength and influence of the sugar
lobby in Washington, DC, as well as their hard and soft money contributions to
political parties. In the past the sugar industry has been quite vocal about the
wording of various dietary guidelines; instead of "eat less sugar," the message
became "choose a diet moderate in sugar."

12. The Healthy Eating Index measured and rated the American eater's own
quality by how little fat he or she consumed. If the eater consumed less than 30%
of his or her daily calories from fat, the eater scored the maximum 10 points.
The study gave no extra points or any fewer points if the eater chose fats from
plant- or animal-based sources.

13. While the Food Guide Pyramid claims that this food group is an "important source of fiber," the examples of starches represented in the pictures at the
base of the pyramid are almost entirely devoid of fiber. There are three loaves of
bread, none of which appear to be whole wheat, a bowl of white rice, a bowl
of white pasta, a picture of saltine crackers, and a bowl of cereal in the shape
of an O. The O's, presumably something similar to the General Mills' Cheerios,
have a scanty 3 grams of fiber per serving.

14. Prior to Renaud and de Lonergil's *Lancet* article, CBS's show *60 Minutes*
aired a story on the "French Paradox" on November 17, 1991. Mike Wallace
was on location in France and reported that despite their fatty diet, the French
maintain one of the lowest rates of heart disease in the world. In a Wall Street
Journal article from January 20, 1992, Kathleen Deveney reported a 45% increase
in wine consumption in the months that followed the CBS broadcast.

Chapter 5. Talking about Taste

1. Of course, there are many cookbooks that employ a discourse of quantification and use science to buttress their recipes. This discourse is most often

found in cookbooks that follow a "diet" plan. For example, Dr. Atkins's *New Diet Revolution* contains recipes that are "controlled carbohydrate" (the bane of the Atkins Diet), and while Atkins's recipes are touted as "delicious," they are "carefully developed by our staff of nutritionists," and each contains nutritional data about the number of carbohydrates, fats, and calories.

2. Traditional techniques often refer to practices that are nearly impossible to capture, like the Italian concept of *quanto basta*, which, roughly translated, means "until it is enough." When making fresh pasta for example, the amount of extra flour you need to finish the pasta during kneading is at the chef's discretion or Q.B.

3. The American ideology that Kennedy feels will "invade" Mexico to its detriment is summarized by American food writer James Villas in *American Taste* (New York: Arbor House, 1982). Villas recognizes America's culinary history, but sees more promise in the future of American cooking: "already our culinary heritage has given us much we can be proud of, and this book is an attempt to celebrate that tradition. But the very legacy demands that within the realm of our experience we act boldly, expand what knowledge we have acquired, use our imagination, and create something truly superior that we can call our own." For Villas, the past is only useful insofar as it becomes the foundation for something better. Here, repeating what was done in the past with greater skill holds no interest for Villas, instead "something truly superior" comes from expanding and inventing, and not preserving or remembering (p. 17). Food that is "authentically American" is not an iteration of the past, but rather a constant search for novelty, which Villas equates with quality.

4. An example of this is the commonly used lipid divisions in Italian cooking. As the climate changes from the top of Italy to the bottom, so too does the lipid of choice in cooking. In the cooler North, close to Slovenia and Austria, pork fat is a common ingredient in cooking. Few cows are raised and the climate does not allow for the successful cultivation of olives. In the middle North of the country, and certainly near the Alpine regions, grazing cows provide sweet and flavorful butter. Thus, much of the fat used in these traditional and regional recipes is butter. Finally, in the South (a region roughly beginning in Tuscany and Emilia-Romagna) the cultivation of olives makes their fragrant oil the selected lipid in most recipes.

5. In Italy, the system of naming regions of wines was drawn up in 1963. Wines are designated DOC, *Denominazione di Origine Controllata*, or DOCG, *Denominazione di Origine Controllata e Garantita*, depending on the region the wine is from. Unlike the French designation of AOC (*Appellation d'Origine Contrôlée*), which is strictly a geographical nomination, the Italian naming system is a place name and a production formula. That is, if a wine's DOC is *Collio*, this means that it is from the Venezia Giulia region, and the grapes have undergone a specified set of processes unique to the wine of that region. French and Italian cheeses also have AOC and DOC designations that too are place names and production formulae.

6. It is not surprising that many of the cookbooks that have such menus or recipes were written before mass transport was available. Transportation technologies

have been both a blessing and a curse to the national diet. While the trucking industry provides tomatoes for Wisconsin in January, it also facilitated the need for a method for picking the tomatoes while they were far from ripe (making them less delicate, but also less flavorful) and inducing ripening with ethylene gas off the vine. As most of us will acknowledge, while we may eat vegetables in the winter, for extra vitamin C to ward off illness for example, the taste of traditional summer vegetables in the winter is watery, bland, and uninspiring.

7. www.chezpanisse.com/pgcommit.html [accessed Nov. 2003] Waters's philosophy, as well as Pellegrino Artusi's and other chefs', may derive from the notion of yin and yang foods of Traditional Chinese Medicine (TCM) or the Indian Ayurveda. In TCM, certain foods are to be eaten at certain times of the year to sustain the body properly and to keep it in rhythm with the seasons and balance the Chinese "vital energy" of *chi* or *qi*. Yang foods, which are warming and sustaining (meats, grains, and long-keeping vegetables like onions, hard squashes, and cabbages) ought to be eaten in the winter months. Yin foods, which are cooling and watery (fresh vegetables and fruits, lighter meats, and fish), ought to be consumed in the summer months to remove heat from the body. While TCM, and Ayurveda do functionalize foods, they do not use quantitative arguments to do so. Instead, there is a sensibility of seasonal opposites—cold-hot, winter-summer—that encourages certain eating patterns.

8. Many of the descriptors have been codified by Ann Noble's *Wine Aroma Wheel*, which categorizes wines' flavors into types: chemical, fruity, woody, earthy, and so forth. Matthew Latkiewicz (2003) points out that the wine wheel is an attempt to "locate our sensation" and to "know" and not merely "experience" wine.

9. Hines, while he may have been the best nationally recognized restaurant reviewer, was not overly concerned with the taste of food. As Harvey Levenstein (1993) argues, Hines represented "the sorry state of American gastronomy" in that his top priority at restaurants was cleanliness, which he often snuck into the kitchen to assess. Because Hines was obsessed with hygiene he often preferred chain restaurants because they were "brightly lit" with "glistening tabletops, and simple food" (pp. 46–47).

10. Unfortunately, many of the restaurant reviews now use a star system to quantify and thus compare. For example, the *New York Times* uses a 0- to 4-star system to rate restaurants, and *Zagat's* uses a 0 to 30 scale to rate the food, décor, and service of the restaurants they review. The French system of Michelin stars, awarding a maximum of 3 stars to the "best" restaurants, began in France in 1900 as the first systematic evaluation of food establishments.

11. I have chosen chowhound.com because it provides the least amount of structural editorial content. The content of chowhound is found in the message boards generated by readers.

12. www.chowhound.com [accessed Dec. 2003] The Chowhound website makes a clear distinction between "foodies" and "Chowhounds." A foodie "eagerly follows food trends" and goes to the restaurants with favorable reviews from the aforementioned restaurant critics. The Chowhound, on the other hand "combs

gleefully through neighborhoods" and "while they appreciate refined ambiance and service, they can't be fooled by mere flash."

13. http://www.chowhound.com/midwest/boards/midwest/messages/13667. html

14. http://www.chowhound.com/midwest/boards/midwest/messages/13682. html

15. http://www.chowhound.com/midwest/boards/midwest/messages/13681. html

16. http://www.chowhound.com/southwest/boards/southwest/messages/10499. html

17. http://www.chowhound.com/southwest/boards/southwest/messages/10523. html

18. http://www.slowfood.com/eng/sf_cose/sf_cose_storia.lasso

19. http://www.slowfood.com/eng/sf_universita/sf_universita.lasso

20. Università di Scienze Gastronomiche promotional pamphlet (p. 7). It is important to note here that the translation of *scienza* from the Italian is not "science" but "knowledge."

21. http://www.slowfood.com/eng/sf_universita/sf_universita.lasso

22. Università di Scienze Gastronomiche promotional pamphlet (p. 8).

23. http://www.slowfood.com/eng/sf_universita/sf_universita.lasso

24. http://www.slowfood.com/eng/sf_master/sf_master_corsi.lasso

25. http://www.slowfood.com/eng/sf_arca_presidi/sf_arca.lasso

26. http://www.slowfood.com/eng/sf_arca_presidi/sf_arca.lasso

27. Carlo Petrini, before founding Slow Food, was a left-wing food and wine journalist with Marxist leanings. His initial foray into politics and food was his organized protest of the McDonald's franchise built near the historic Spanish Steps in Rome.

References

An act to establish a Department of Agriculture, Chapter 72, Bill 249, 37th Congress, Session 2, May 15, 1862.

Anderson, E. N. 2005. *Everyone eats: Understanding food and culture.* New York: New York University Press.

Apple, Rima. 1995. Science gendered: Nutrition in the United States, 1840–1940. In *The science and culture of nutrition 1840–1940,* eds. Harmke Kamminga and Andrew Cunningham, pp. 129–154. Atlanta, GA: Editions Rodopi.

Apple, Rima. 2006. *Perfect motherhood: Science and childrearing in America.* New Brunswick, NJ: Rutgers University Press.

Artusi, Pellegrino. 1996. *The art of eating well.* Trans. Kyle Phillips III. New York: Random House.

Ashby, Sir Eric. 1959. *Technology and the academics: An essay on universities and the scientific revolution.* New York: MacMillan.

Atkinson, Edward. 1886–1887. The food question in America and Europe. *Century Magazine* 33, pp. 238–248.

Atkinson, Edward. 1886–1887. The margins of profits. *Century Magazine,* 33, pp. 923–931.

Atkinson, Edward. 1886–1887. The relative strength and weakness of nations. *Century Magazine* 33, pp. 423–435 and pp. 613–621.

Atwater, Wilbur O. 1876. U.S. Department of Agriculture, Agricultural-experiment stations in Europe. *Report of the Commissioner of Agriculture for the Year 1875.* Washington, DC: Government Printing Office.

Atwater, Wilbur O. 1878. On the quantitative determination of fats. *Proceeding of the American Chemical Society* 2, pp. 84–98.

Atwater, Wilbur O. 1887a. Food, how it nourishes the body. *Century Magazine,* 34, pp. 237–251.

Atwater, Wilbur O. 1887b. The chemistry of food and nutrition. *Century Magazine,* 34, pp. 59–74.

Atwater, Wilbur O. 1887c. The digestibility of food. *Century Magazine,* 34, pp. 733–739.

Atwater, Wilbur O. 1887d. The potential energy of food. *Century Magazine,* 34, pp. 397–405.

Atwater, Wilbur O. 1889. U.S. Department of Agriculture, *Report of the director of the Office of Experiment Stations for 1889.* Washington, DC: Government Printing Office.

Atwater, Wilbur O. 1890. U.S. Department of Agriculture, *Report of the director of the Office of Experiment Stations for 1890.* Washington, DC: Government Printing Office.

Atwater, Wilbur. 1893. U.S. Department of Agriculture, Suggestions for the establishment of food laboratories in connection with the agricultural experiment stations of the United States. *Office of Experiment Stations Bulletin*, no. 17. Washington, DC: Government Printing Office.

Atwater, Wilbur O. 1895. U.S. Department of Agriculture, Food and diet. *1894 Yearbook of Agriculture.* Washington, DC: Government Printing Office.

Atwater, Wilbur O. 1896. U.S. Department of Agriculture, The chemical composition of American food materials. *Office of Experiment Stations Bulletin*, no. 28. Washington, DC: Government Printing Office.

Atwater, Wilbur O. 1902. U.S. Department of Agriculture, Principles of nutrition and nutritive value of food. *Farmers' Bulletin*, no. 142. Washington, DC: Government Printing Office.

Atwater, Wilbur O., and E. B. Rosa. 1899. U.S. Department of Agriculture, Description of a new respiration calorimeter and experiments on the conservation of energy in the human body. *Office of Experiment Stations Bulletin*, no. 63. Washington, DC: Government Printing Office.

Balogh, Brian. 1991. *Chain reaction: Expert debate and public participation in American commercial nuclear power, 1945–1975.* New York: Cambridge University Press.

Bastianich, Joseph, and David Lynch. 2002. *Vino Italiano: The regional wines of Italy.* New York: Clarkson-Potter.

Bazerman, Charles. 1988. *Shaping written knowledge: The genre and activity of the experimental article in science.* Madison: University of Wisconsin Press.

Beardsworth, Alan, and Teresa Keil. 1997. *Sociology on the menu: An invitation to the study of food and society.* New York: Routledge.

Belasco, Warren. 1993. *Appetite for change: How the counterculture took on the food industry.* Ithaca, NY: Cornell University Press.

Belasco, Warren. 1997. Food, morality and social reform. In *Morality and health*, eds. Allan Brandt and Paul Rozin, pp. 185–200. New York: Routledge.

Belasco, Warren. 2006. *Meals to come: A history of the future of food.* Berkeley, CA: University of California Press.

Bell, Daniel. 1973. *The coming of post-industrial society: A venture in social forecasting.* New York: Basic Books.

Bentley, Amy. 1998. *Eating for victory: Food rationing and the politics of domesticity.* Urbana: University of Illinois Press.

Bloor, D. 1991. *Knowledge and social imagery* (2nd ed.). London: University of Chicago Press.

Bogo, Jennifer. 2002. Hungry for change: Chef Alice Waters is convinced that the path to awakening students' minds to their environment is through their stomachs, so she's helped build them a schoolyard—and make it edible. *Audubon*, 104, March–April, p. 30.

Boyd, William, and Michael Watts. 1997. Agro-industrial just-in-time: The chicken industry and postwar american capitalism. In *Globalising food: Agrarian questions and global restructuring*, eds. David Goodman and Michael Watts, pp. 192–225. New York: Routledge.

Brenner, Leslie. 2000. *American appetite: The coming of age of a national cuisine*. New York: HarperCollins Books.

Brown, Cheryl. 2002. Consumers' preference for locally produced food: A study in southeast Missouri. *American Journal of Alternative Agriculture*, 9, p. 3.

Browne, William. 1988. *Private interests, public policy, and American agriculture*. Lawrence: University Press of Kansas.

Browne, William. 1995. *Cultivating Congress: Constituents, issues, and agricultural policymaking*. Lawrence: University Press of Kansas.

Brownlee, Shannon, and Robert Barnett. 1994, July. A loaf of bread, a glass of wine. *U.S. News and World Report*, 4, p. 62.

Buchanan, Richard. 2001. Design and the new rhetoric: Productive arts in the philosophy of culture. *Philosophy and Rhetoric*, 34, pp. 183–206.

Burros, Marian. 1991, April 10. Rethink 4 food groups, doctors tell U.S. *New York Times*, p. C1.

Burros, Marian. 1991, May 8. Are cattlemen now guarding the henhouse? *New York Times*, p. C1.

Callahan, Maureen. 2003, April. Eyes on the size. *Cooking Light*, pp. 68–72.

Campos, Paul. 2004. *The obesity myth: Why America's obsession with weight is hazardous to your health*. New York: Gotham Books.

Carpenter, Kenneth. 1986. *The history of scurvy and vitamin C*. New York: Cambridge University Press.

Carpenter, Kenneth J. 1994. The life and times of W. O. Atwater (1844–1907). *The Journal of Nutrition*, 124, pp. 1707S–1714S.

Child, Julia, Louisette Bertholle, and Simone Beck. 1966. *Mastering the art of French cooking*. New York: Alfred A Knopf.

Cochrane, Willard W. 1993. *Development of American agriculture: A historical analysis* (2nd ed.). Minneapolis: University of Minnesota Press.

Cohen, I. Bernard. 1963. Science in America: The nineteenth century. In *Paths of American thought*, eds. Arthur Schlesinger Jr. and Morton White, pp. 167–189. Boston: Houghton-Mifflin.

Cohen, Lizabeth. 1991. *Making a new deal: Industrial workers in Chicago, 1919–1939*. New York: Cambridge University Press.

Cohen, Patricia C. 1999. *A calculating people: The spread of numeracy in early America*. New York: Routledge.

Combs, G. 1994. Celebration of the past: Nutrition at the USDA. *The Journal of Nutrition*, 124, p. 1729S.

Conigrave, K. M. et al. 2001. A prospective study of drinking patterns in relation to risk of type 2 diabetes among men. *Diabetes*, 50, 10, pp. 2390–2395.

Cornwall, E. E. 1916. The treatment of obesity by a rational diet. *Boston Medical and Surgical Journal* 175, 17, pp. 601–602.

Counihan, Carole, ed. 2002. *Food in the U.S.A.: A reader*. New York: Routledge.

Counihan, Carole, and Penny van Esterik, eds. 1997. *Food and culture: A reader*. New York: Routledge.

Cowan, Ruth. 1983. *More work for mother.* New York: Basic Books.

Cravens, Hamilton. 1990. Establishing the science of nutrition at the USDA: Ellen Swallow Richards and her allies. *Agricultural History,* 64, pp. 122–133.

Cravens, Hamilton. 1996. The German-American science of racial nutrition. In *Technical knowledge in American culture: Science, technology and medicine since the early 1800's,* eds. Hamilton Cravens, A. Marcus, and D. Katzman, pp. 125–148. Tuscaloosa: University of Alabama Press.

Critser, Greg. 2003. *Fat land: How Americans became the fattest people in the world.* New York: Houghton-Mifflin.

Cronin F. J., A. M. Shaw et al. 1987. Developing a food guidance system to implement the dietary guidelines. *Journal of Nutrition Education,* 19, pp. 281–302.

Crosby, Alfred. 1997. *The measure of reality: Quantification and the Western world, 1250–1600.* New York: Cambridge University Press.

Curtin, Deane, and Lisa Heldke. 1992. *Cooking, eating, thinking: Transformative philosophies of food.* Bloomington, IN: Indiana University Press.

Danbom, David. 1986. The agricultural experiment station and professionalization: Scientists' goals for agriculture. *Agricultural History,* 60, pp. 246–255.

Daniels, George H. 1968. *American science in the age of Jackson.* New York: Columbia University Press.

Davis, Joseph S. 1932. The specter of dearth of food: History's answer to Sir William Crookes. In *Facts and factors in economic history.* Cambridge, MA: Harvard University Press.

De La Peña, Carolyn. 2003. *The body electric: How strange machines built the modern American.* New York: New York University Press.

Dettwyler, Katherine. 1994. *Dancing skeletons: Life and death in West Africa.* Prospect Heights, IL: Waveland.

Deveney, Kathleen. 1992, January 20. America is taking heart healthy habits from France. *Wall Street Journal,* 20, p. B7.

Dickson, David. 1984. *The new politics of science.* Chicago: University of Chicago Press.

Dolby, Virginia. 1998, May. The surprising benefits of moderate wine consumption. *Better Nutrition,* 60, p. 16.

Douglas, Mary. 1984. *Food in the social order: Studies in food and festivities in three American communities.* New York: Russell Sage Foundation.

Du Bois, Cora. 1941. Attitudes toward food and hunger in Alor. In *Language, culture, and personality,* eds. Leslie Spier et. al., pp. 272–281. Menasha, WI: Sapir Memorial Publication Fund.

Duffy, John. 1990. *The sanitarians: A history of American public health.* Urbana, IL: University of Illinois Press.

Dupree, A. Hunter. 1957. *Science in the federal government: A history of policies and activities to 1940.* Cambridge: Belknap Press.

Dupree, A. Hunter. 1963. Central scientific organization in the United States government. *Minerva,* pp. 457–458.

Dyson, Lowell K. 2000, January–April. American cuisine in the 20th century. *Food Review,* 23, p. 5.

Engelhardt, Elizabeth. 2001. Beating biscuits in Appalachia: Race, class, and gender politics of women baking bread. In *Cooking lessons: The politics and gender of food*, ed. Sherrie Inness, pp. 151–168. Lanham: Rowman and Littlefield.

Eskin, Leah. 1998, July–August. State fair. *Saveur*, 28, p. 45.

Fahnestock, Jeanne. 1999. *Rhetorical figures in science*. New York: Oxford University Press.

Ferleger, Lou. 1990a. Uplifting American agriculture: Experiment station scientists and the Office of Experiment Stations in the early years after the Hatch Act. *Agricultural History*, 64, p. 11.

Ferleger, Lou, ed. 1990b. *Agriculture and national development: Views on the nineteenth century*. Ames: Iowa State University Press.

Firth, Raymond. 1934. The sociological study of native diet. In *Africa*, 7, pp. 401–414.

Fleck, Ludwik. 1979. *The genesis and development of a scientific fact*. Chicago: University of Chicago Press.

Floyd, Janet, and Laurel Forster. 2003. *The recipe reader: Narratives, contexts and traditions*. Burlington, VT: Ashgate Publishing.

Food and Drug Administration Publication, 21 CFR Part 101, "Food Labeling: Nutrient Content Claims, General Principles; Health Claims, General Requirements and Other Specific Requirements for Individual Health Claims" Docket 94P-0390, p. 66208.

Fortes, Myer, and S. L. Fortes. 1936. Food in the domestic economy of Tallensi. *Africa*, 9, pp. 237–276.

Foucault, Michel. 1994. *The birth of the clinic: An archaeology of medical perception*. New York: Vintage Books.

Fowler, Bertram B. 1942. *Food, a weapon for victory*. Boston: Little, Brown and Company.

Frängsmyr, Tore, ed. 1990. *The quantifying spirit in the 18th century*. Berkeley: University of California Press.

Friedson, Elliot. 1984. Are professions necessary? In *The authority of experts: Studies in history and theory*, ed. Thomas Haskell, pp. 3–27. Bloomington: Indiana University Press.

Fuller, Steve. 1988. *Social epistemology*. Bloomington: Indiana University Press.

Funes, Fernando et al. 2002. *Sustainable agriculture and resistance*. New York: Food First Books.

Galambos, Louis. 1982. *America at middle age: A new history of the United States in the twentieth century*. New York: McGraw-Hill.

Galer-Unti, Regina. 1995. *Hunger and food assistance policy in the United States*. New York: Garland Publishing.

Gard, Michael, and Jan Wright. 2005. *The obesity epidemic: Science, morality, and ideology*. New York: Routledge.

Gates, Paul W. 1965. *Agriculture and the Civil War*. New York: Alfred A. Knopf.

Geiger, Roger. 2004. *To advance knowledge: The growth of American research universities, 1900–1940*. Edison, NJ: Transaction.

Gladwell, Malcolm. 1991, April 13. U.S. rethinks, redraws the food groups. *Washington Post*, p. A1.

Gladwell, Malcolm. 1992, April 28. The $855,000 pyramid; U.S. revises nutritional guidelines chart. *Washington Post*, p. A1.

Gladwell, Malcolm. 1992, May 12. USDA's warmed-over food pyramid. *Washington Post*, p. D20.

Gold, Rozanne. 2003, January. For Super Bowl, a super party. *Bon Appetit*, p. 43.

Goldberg, Shoshana. 2002, September/October. Braided bread. *Saveur*, 61, p. 41.

Goodman, David, and Michael Redclift. 1991. *Refashioning nature: Food, ecology and culture*. New York: Routledge.

Goodman, David, and Michael Watts, eds. 1997. *Globalising food: Agrarian questions and global restructuring*. New York: Routledge.

Gratzer, Walter. 2005. *Terrors of the table: The curious history of nutrition*. New York: Oxford University Press.

Graves, Heather. 2005. *Rhetoric in(to) science: Style as invention in inquiry*. Cresskill, NJ: Hampton Press.

Grønbæk, M. et al. 2000. Type of alcohol consumed and mortality from all causes, coronary heart disease, and cancer. *Annals of Internal Medicine*, 133, 6, pp. 411–419.

Gross, Alan G. 1996. *The rhetoric of science*. London: Harvard University Press.

Gross, Alan. 2006. *Starring the text: The place of rhetoric in science studies*. Carbondale, IL: Southern Illinois University Press, 2006.

Gross, Alan, and William Keith. 1997. *Rhetorical hermeneutics: Invention and interpretation in the age of science*. Albany: State University of New York Press.

Guither, Harold D. 1980. *The food lobbyists*. Lexington, MA: Lexington Books.

Hacking, Ian. 1983. *Representing and intervening: Introductory topics in the philosophy of natural science*. New York: Cambridge University Press.

Hacking, Ian. 1990. *The taming of chance*. Cambridge: Cambridge University Press.

Hackman, Robert. 1998, September. Flavinoids and the French paradox. *USA Today*, 127, pp. 58–60.

Hadwiger, Don, and William Browne. 1978. *The new politics of food*. Lexington, MA: Lexington Books.

Halliday, M. A. K., and J. R. Martin. 1993. *Writing science: Literacy and discursive power*. Pittsburgh: University of Pittsburgh Press.

Halweil, Brian. 2003, May 1 and 2. The rise of food democracy. *The Snail*, p. 8.

Hankins, Thomas L., and Robert J. Silverman. 1995. *Instruments and the imagination*. Princeton: Princeton University Press.

Harding, T. Swann. 1947. *Two blades of grass: A history of scientific development in the U.S. Department of Agriculture*. Norman: University of Oklahoma Press.

Hargreaves, Sally. 2000. Researchers get closer to understanding "French paradox." *The Lancet*, 356, p. 139.

Haskell, Thomas. 1984. Are professions necessary? In *The authority of experts*, ed. Thomas Haskell, pp. 28–83. Bloomington: Indiana University Press.

Haskell, Thomas. 2000. *The emergence of professional social science: The American Social Science Association and the nineteenth-century crisis of authority*. Baltimore: Johns Hopkins University Press.

Hatch Act 1887, Section 3, Chapter 314, 49th Congress, Session 2, March 2, 1887.

Hauser, Gerard. 2002. *Introduction to rhetorical theory*. Prospect Heights: Waveland Press.

Hazan, Marcella. 2000. *Essentials of classic Italian cooking*. New York: Alfred A. Knopf.

Heldke, Lisa. 2003. *Exotic appetites: Ruminations of a food adventurer*. New York: Routledge.

Herrick, James. 1998. *The history and theory of rhetoric: An introduction*. Boston: Allyn and Bacon.

Hesser, Amanda. 2003, July 26. Endangered species: Slow food, interview with Carlo Petrini. *New York Times*, p. B9.

Hirsheimer, Christopher. 2000, September/October. Belles. *Saveur*, 45, pp. 90–95.

Hollinger, David. 1984. Inquiry and uplift: Late nineteenth-century American academics and the moral efficiency of scientific practice. In *The authority of experts: Historical and theoretical essays*, ed. Thomas Haskell, pp. 142–156. Bloomington: Indiana University Press.

Holmes-McNary, M., et al. 2000. Chemopreventative properties of trans-resveratrol are associated with inhibition of activation of the IkappaB kinase. *Cancer Research*, 60, pp. 3477–3483.

Hoy, Suellen. 1995. *Chasing dirt: The American pursuit of cleanliness*. New York: Oxford University Press.

Hunt, Caroline. 1917. U.S. Department of Agriculture, *How to Select Foods Bulletin*, no. 808. Washington, DC: Government Printing Office.

Jefford, Andrew. 2000. *Wine tastes wine styles*. London: Ryland, Peters and Small.

Jenkins, Steve. 1996. *The cheese primer*. New York: Workman Publishing.

Johnson, Hugh. 1999. *Hugh Johnson's how to enjoy your wine*. New York: Simon and Schuster.

Jones, Evan. 1981. 2nd ed. *American food: The gastronomic story*. New York: Vintage Books.

Kahn, Miriam. 1986. *Always hungry, never greedy: Food and the expression of gender in a Melanesian society*. New York: Cambridge University Press.

Kalins, Dorothy. 1997, September/October. Mean cuisine. *Saveur*, 21, p. 16.

Kamminga, Harmke, and Andrew Cunningham. 1995. *The science and culture of nutrition, 1840–1940*. Atlanta, GA: Editions Rodopi B.V.

Kantor, Linda S. 1996, January–April. Many Americans are not meeting Food Guide Pyramid dietary recommendations. *Food Review*, p. 3.

Kennedy, Diana. 1998. *My Mexico*. New York: Clarkson Potter.

Kimbell, Andrew. 2002. *Fatal harvest: The tragedy of industrial agriculture*. New York: Island Press.

Kirkendall, Richard S. 1966. *Social scientists and farm politics in the age of Roosevelt.* Columbia: University of Missouri Press.

Kirkendall, Richard S. 1975. The New Deal and agriculture. *The New Deal, Volume 1,* eds. John Braeman, Robert Bremner, and David Brody. Columbus: Ohio University Press.

Kuhn, Thomas. 1996. *The structure of scientific revolutions.* Chicago: University of Chicago Press.

Kula, Witold. 1986. *Measures and men.* Trans. R. Szreter. Princeton: Princeton University Press.

LaFollette, Marcelle C. 1990. *Making science our own: Public images of science.* Chicago: University of Chicago Press.

Lamb Hayes, Joanne. 2000. *Grandma's wartime kitchen: World War II and the way we cooked.* New York: St. Martin's Press.

Larkin, M. 1999. U.S. Food and Drug Administration, Ways to win at weight loss. In *FDA Consumer.* Washington, DC: Government Printing Office.

Latkiewicz, Matthew. 2003, Fall. Notes from a wine-tasting, being an inquiry into sensation. *Gastronomica* 4, pp. 42–45.

Latour, Bruno, and Steve Woolgar. 1986. *Laboratory life: The construction of scientific facts.* Princeton: Princeton University Press.

Lebow, R. N. 2006. Robert S. McNamara: Max Weber's nightmare. *International Relations* 20, pp. 211–224.

Leidner, Robin. 1993. *Fast food, fast talk: Service work and the routinization of everyday life.* Berkeley: University of California Press.

Leonardi, Susan. 1989. Recipes for reading: Summer pasta, lobster à la Riseholme, and Key lime pie. *PMLA* 104, pp. 340–347.

Levenstein, Harvey. 1993. *Paradox of plenty: A social history of eating in modern America.* New York: Oxford University Press.

Levenstein, Harvey. 2003. *Revolution at the table: The transformation of the American diet.* Berkeley: University of California Press.

Lewis, Edna. 1988. *In pursuit of flavor.* New York: Alfred A. Knopf.

Liebig, Justus. 1842. *Animal chemistry, or organic chemistry in its application to physiology and pathology.* Cambridge: John Owen.

Lupton, Deborah. 1996. *Food, the body and the self.* Thousand Oaks, CA: Sage Publications.

Macbeth, Helen, and Jeremy MacClancy, eds. 2004. *Researching food habits: Methods and Problems.* New York: Bergham Books.

Madison, Deborah. 2002. *Local flavors: Cooking and eating from America's farmers' markets.* New York: Broadway Books.

Marling, Karal Ann. 1992. *As seen on TV: The visual culture of everyday life in the 1950s.* Chicago: University of Chicago Press.

Mars, Valerie. 1994. A la Russe: The new way of dining. In *Luncheon, nuncheon and other meals: Eating with the Victorians,* ed. Anne Wilson, pp. 117–144. Stroud: Alan Sutton.

Maynard, J. 1962. Wilbur O. Atwater: A biographical sketch. *Journal of Nutrition* 78, pp. 1–9.

McCloskey, Deirdre. 1998. *The rhetoric of economics*. Madison: University of Wisconsin Press.

McCollum, Elmer. 1957. *A history of nutrition: The sequence of ideas in nutrition investigations*. Boston: Houghton Mifflin.

Mcelvaine, Robert. 1993. *The Great Depression: America 1929–1941*. Pittsburgh: Three Rivers Press.

McInerny, Jay. 2002. *Bacchus and me*. New York: Vintage Books.

McIntosh, Alex. 1996. *Sociologies of food and nutrition*. New York: Plenum Press.

McIntosh, Elaine. 1995. *American food habits in historical perspective*. Westport, CT: Praeger Publishing.

McKibben, Bill. 2003, December. Small world. *Harper's Magazine*, p. 54.

McWilliams, James. 2005. *A revolution in eating: How the quest for food shaped America*. New York: Columbia University Press.

Meigs, Anna. 1984. *Food, sex, and pollution: A New Guinea religion*. New Brunswick, NJ: Rutgers University Press.

Menninger, Karl. 1969. *Number words and number symbols: A cultural history of numbers*. Trans. Paul Broneer. Cambridge: MIT Press.

Merton, Robert K. 1974. *The sociology of science: Theoretical and empirical investigations*. Chicago: University of Chicago Press.

Miller, Michael. 1994, June 17. Call for a daily dose of wine ferments critics. *Wall Street Journal*, p. B1.

Miller, Toby. 1993. *The well-tempered self: Citizenship, culture and the postmodern subject*. Baltimore: Johns Hopkins University Press.

Mintz, Sidney. 1985. *Sweetness and power*. New York: Penguin.

Mintz, Sidney. 1997. Sugar and morality. In *Morality and health*, eds. Allan Brandt and Paul Rozin, pp. 173–184. New York: Routledge.

Mokdad, Ali H. et al. 1999. The spread of the obesity epidemic in the United States, 1991–1998. *Journal of the American Medical Association*, 282, pp. 1519–1522.

Montgomery, Scott L. 1996. *The scientific voice*. New York: Guilford Press.

Munson, M., and Yeykal, T. 1996, March. Doctor's wine list: Which selections your heart might like. *Prevention*, 48, pp. 32–34.

Nabhan, Gary. 2002. *Coming home to eat: The pleasures and politics of local foods*. New York: W. W. Norton.

Nelson, John, Alan Megill, and Donald McCloskey. 1987. *The rhetoric of the human science: Language and argument in scholarship and public affairs*. Madison: University of Wisconsin Press.

Nestle, Marion, and Michael Jacobson. 2000, January/February. Halting the obesity epidemic: A public health policy approach. *Public Health Reports*, 115, pp. 12–24.

Nestle, Marion. 2002. *Food politics: How the food industry influences nutrition and health*. Berkeley: University of California Press.

Newman, Frank J. 1981. The era of expertise: The growth, the spread, and ultimately the decline of the national commitment to the concept of the highly trained expert: 1945–1970. PhD dissertation, Stanford University.

Nichols, Buford. 1994. Atwater and USDA nutrition research and service: A prologue of the past century. *Journal of Nutrition*, 124, pp. 1718S–1729S.

Nixon, Russell, and Paul Samuelson. 1940. Estimates of Unemployment in the United States. *Review of Economic Statistics*, 22, pp. 106–107.

Office of War Information. 1942, December 27. *Food rationing and the war*—An address by Mr. Elmer Davis. Washington, DC: Government Printing Office.

Oldways Preservation and Exchange Trust. 2001. Retrieved February 28, 2001 http://www.oldwayspt.org/html/p_med_com.htm. Boston: Oldways.

Oldways Preservation and Exchange Trust. 1994. *1994 international conference on the Mediterranean diet: Notes accompanying release of the official healthy traditional Mediterranean diet pyramid.* San Francisco: Oldways.

Oleson, Alexandra, and John Voss. 1979. *The organization of knowledge in modern America, 1860–1920.* Baltimore: Johns Hopkins University Press.

Oliver, J. Eric. 2006. *Fat politics: The real story behind America's obesity epidemic.* New York: Oxford University Press.

Ortony, Andrew. 1993. *Metaphor and thought.* New York: Cambridge University Press.

Page, Esther, and Louise Phipard. 1956. U.S. Department of Agriculture, *Essentials of an adequate diet*, bulletin no. 160. Washington, DC: Government Printing Office.

Parker-Pope, Tara. 2003, May 20. Eating for six? That pasta primavera has far more "servings" than you think. *Wall Street Journal*, p. D1.

Paumgarten, Nick. 2003, December 22–29. Tables for two. *New Yorker*, p. 25.

Peele, Stanton. 1999, October 31. Bottle battle. *Reason*, 31, p. 52.

Pennington, A. W. 1954. Treatment of obesity: Developments of the past 150 years. *American Journal of Digestive Diseases*, 21, pp. 65–69.

Pera, Marcello. 1994. *The discourses of science.* Chicago: University of Chicago Press.

Perelman, Chaim, and L. Olbrechts-Tyteca. 1969. *The new rhetoric: A treatise on argumentation.* South Bend, IN: University of Notre Dame Press.

Peters, John Durham. 2005. *Courting the abyss: Free speech and the liberal tradition.* Chicago: University of Chicago Press.

Pollan, Michael. 2003, May/June. Cruising on the ark of taste. *Mother Jones Magazine*, pp. 74–75.

Pollan, Michael. 2006. *The omnivore's dilemma.* New York: Penguin.

Pollan, Michael. 2008. *In defense of food: An eater's manifesto.* New York: Penguin.

Pollock, Nancy. 1992. *These roots remain: Food habits in islands of the central and eastern Pacific since Western contact.* Honolulu: Institute for Polynesian Studies.

Porter, Theodore. 1986. *The rise of statistical thinking 1820–1900.* Princeton: Princeton University Press.

Porter, Theodore. 1995. *Trust in numbers: The pursuit of objectivity in science and public life.* Princeton: Princeton University Press.

Prial, Frank. 2002, September 18. Wines of the times: Getting it right in the Rhone. *New York Times*, p. F10.

Price, Don K. 1965. *The scientific estate.* Cambridge, MA: Harvard University Press.

Rabinbach, Anson. 1990. *The human motor: Energy, fatigue and the origins of modernity.* New York: Basic Books.

Raver, Anne. 2001, December 2. Hunting, gathering, growing in the 21st century. *New York Times*, p. 14.

Reardon, Joan. 1994. *M. F. K. Fisher, Julia Child and Alice Waters: Celebrating the pleasures of the table.* New York: Harmony Books.

Reichl, Ruth. 1999, November. So much for tradition. *Gourmet*, p. 28.

Reichl, Ruth. 2001, November. Holiday promise. *Gourmet*, p. 18.

Reichl, Ruth. 2003, November. Rehearsal dinners. *Gourmet*, p. 20.

Reingold, Nathan. 1976. Definitions and speculations: The professionalization of science in America in the nineteenth century. *The pursuit of knowledge in the early American republic*, eds. Alexandra Oleson and Sanborn Brown, pp. 33–69. Baltimore: Johns Hopkins University Press.

Reiter, Esther. 1991. *Making fast food: From the frying pan into the fryer.* Montreal: McGill-Queen's University Press.

Renaud, Serge, and M. de Lorgeril. 1992. Wine alcohol, platelets, and the French paradox for coronary heart disease. *The Lancet*, 339, pp. 1523–1526.

Reynolds, C. V. 1993, January. Wining and dining. *Discover*, p. 46.

Richards, Audrey. 1932. *Hunger and work in a savage tribe.* London: Routledge.

Ritzer, George. 1993. *The McDonaldization of society.* Thousand Oaks, CA: Pine Forge Press.

Roe, Daphne. 1973. *A plague of corn: The social history of pellagra.* Ithaca: Cornell University Press.

Root, Waverly, and Richard de Rochemont. 1976. *Eating in America.* New York: William Morrow.

Rosenberg, Charles E. 1976. *No other gods: On science and American social life.* Baltimore: Johns Hopkins University Press.

Rosenberg, Charles E. 1977. Rationalization and reality in the shaping of American agricultural research, 1875–1914. *Social Studies of Science*, 7, p. 403.

Rourke, Francis E. 1969. *Bureaucracy, politics, and public policy.* Boston: Little, Brown.

Sack, Daniel. 2000. *Whitebread Protestants: Food and religion in American culture.* New York: St. Martin's Press.

Saloutos, Theodore. 1974. New Deal agricultural policy: An evaluation. *Journal of American History*, 61, pp. 394–416.

Saloutos, Theodore. 1982. *The American farmers and the New Deal.* Ames: Iowa State University Press.

Sarfatti Larson, Magali. 1984. Expertise and expert power. In *The authority of experts*, ed. Thomas Haskell, pp. 28–83. Bloomington: Indiana University Press.

Satcher, David. 2001. U.S. Department of Health and Human Services, Office of the Surgeon General, *Call to action to prevent and decrease overweight and obesity 2001.* Washington, DC: Government Printing Office.

Savage, James. 1999. *Funding science in America: Congress, universities, and the politics of the academic pork barrel.* New York: Cambridge University Press.

Schlesinger Jr., Arthur. 1958. *The coming of the New Deal*. Boston: Houghton Mifflin.

Schlesinger Jr., Arthur. 1960. *The politics of upheaval*. Boston: Houghton Mifflin.

Schlesinger Jr., Arthur, and Morton White, eds. 1963. *Paths of American thought*. Boston: Houghton Mifflin.

Scholten, Paul. 1989. Wine and health. *Wines and Vines*, 70, pp. 13–16.

Schudson, Michael. 1999. *The good citizen: A history of American civic life*. Cambridge: Harvard University Press.

Schwartz-Nobel, Loretta. 2002. *Growing up empty: The hunger epidemic in America*. New York: Harper Collins.

Scrinis, Gyorgy. 2008. On the ideology of nutritionism. *Gastronomica*, 8, 39–48.

Seigneur, M., J. Bonnet, B. Dorian, et al. 1990. Effect of alcohol, white wine and red wine on platelet function and serum lipids. *Journal of Applied Cardiology*, 5, pp. 215–222.

Sentate Resolution 291 Report No. 1416, July 30, 1968, 90th Congresss, 2nd Session.

Shapiro, Laura. 2001. *Perfection salad: Women and cooking at the turn of the century*. New York: Modern Library.

Shorto, Russell. 2004, January 11. A short-order revolutionary. *New York Times Magazine*, pp. 18–21.

Sinclair, Upton. 1981. *The jungle*. New York: Bantam Books.

Spigel, Lynn. 1992. *Make room for TV: Television and the family ideal in postwar America*. Chicago: University of Chicago Press.

Stacey, Michelle. 1994. *Consumed: Why Americans love, hate and fear food*. New York: Simon and Schuster.

Stampfer, M. et al. 2005. Effects of moderate alcohol consumption on cognitive function in women. *New England Journal of Medicine*, 352, 3, pp. 245–253.

Starr, Paul. 1982. *The social transformation of American medicine*. New York: Basic Books.

Stern, Jane, and Michael Stern. 2003, July. Nuts for the Northwest. *Gourmet*, pp. 54–55.

Stiebeling, Hazel. 1933. U.S. Department of Agriculture, *Diets at four levels of nutritive content and cost*, circular no. 296. Washington, DC: Government Printing Office.

Telfer, Elizabeth. 1996. *Food for thought: Philosophy and food*. New York: Routledge.

Theophano, Janet. 2002. *Eat my words*. New York: Palgrave.

Thomas, Patricia. 1994, March. A toast to the heart. *Harvard Health Letter*, pp. 4–5.

Tomes, Nancy. 1998. *The gospel of germs: Men, women and the microbe in American life*. Cambridge, MA: Harvard University Press. pp. 91–113.

Trager, James. 1995. *The food chronology*. New York: Henry Holt and Company.

True, Alfred C. 1937. *A history of agricultural experimentation and research in the United States 1607–1925*. Washington, DC: Government Printing Office.

U.S. Bureau of Alcohol, Tobacco and Firearms. 1999, February 5. *Treasury News.* Washington, DC: Government Printing Office.

U.S. Department of Agriculture. 1889. *Report of the Director of the Office of Experiment Stations for 1889.* Washington, DC: Government Printing Office.

U.S. Department of Agriculture. 1890. *Report of the Director of the Office of Experiment Stations for 1890.* Washington, DC: Government Printing Office.

U.S. Department of Agriculture. 1900. *Remarks of M. H. Buckam, proceedings of the thirteenth annual convention of the Association of American Agricultural Colleges and Experiment Stations, held at San Francisco, CA, July 5–6, 1899. Office of Experiment Stations Bulletin,* no. 76. Washington, DC: Government Printing Office.

U.S. Department of Agriculture. 1941. *Yardstick for good nutrition.* Washington, DC: Government Printing Office.

U.S. Department of Agriculture. 1943, July (revised). *National wartime food guide,* NFC-4. Washington, DC: Government Printing Office.

U.S. Department of Agriculture. 1946. *Basic seven.* Leaflet 288. Washington, DC: Government Printing Office

U.S. Department of Agriculture. 1963. *A century of service: The first hundred years of the United States Department of Agriculture.* Washington, DC: Government Printing Office.

U.S. Department of Agriculture. 1969. *Hearings before the select committee on nutrition and human needs and the United States Senate, part 1: Problems and prospects.* Washington, DC: Government Printing Office.

U.S. Department of Agriculture. 1976. *Legislative history of the select committee on nutrition and human needs.* Washington, DC: Government Printing Office.

U.S. Department of Agriculture. 1977, December. *Dietary goals for the United States,* 2nd ed. Washington, DC: Government Printing Office.

U.S. Department of Agriculture. 1977. *Hearings of the 64th select committee on nutrition and human needs of the U.S. Senate, 95th congress, 1st session, part 1: Cardiovascular disease, February 1–2, 1977.* Washington, DC: Government Printing Office.

U.S. Department of Agriculture. 1980. *The hassle-free guide to a better diet.* Leaflet 567. Washington, DC: Government Printing Office

U.S. Department of Agriculture. 1992, revised 1996. The food guide pyramid. *USDA Home and Garden Bulletin,* no. 252. Washington, DC: Government Printing Office.

U.S. Department of Agriculture. 1993. September. Human Nutrition Information Service, *USDA's food guide: Background and development,* miscellaneous publication no. 1514. Washington, DC: Government Printing Office.

U.S. Department of Agriculture. 1994–1996, October. Center for Nutrition Policy and Promotion, *The healthy eating index.* Washington, DC: Government Printing Office.

U.S. Department of Agriculture. 1995. *Nutrition and your health: Dietary guidelines for Americans.* Home and Garden Bulletin 232. Washington, DC: Government Printing Office.

U.S. Department of Agriculture. 1999. Food portions and servings, how do they differ? *Nutrition Insights*, 11, Washington, DC: Government Printing Office.

U.S. Department of Agriculture. 2000. Serving sizes in the food guide pyramid and on the nutrition facts label: What's different and why? *Nutrition Insights*, 22, USDA and CNPP. Washington, DC: Government Printing Office.

U.S. Department of Agriculture. 2002. How much are you eating? *USDA Home and Garden Bulletin*, no. 267. Washington, DC: Government Printing Office.

U.S. Department of Agriculture. 2003. FR Part 68 No. 176, Centre for Nutrition Policy and Promotion; Notice of Availability of Proposed Food Guide Pyramid Daily Food Intake Patterns and Technical Support Data and Announcement of Public Comment Period. p. 53539.

U.S. Department of Agriculture. 2005. *Dietary guidelines for Americans*. Washington, DC: Government Printing Office.

U.S. Department of Health, Education and Welfare. 1980. *Nutrition and your health: Dietary guidelines for Americans*. Washington, DC: Government Printing Office.

U.S. Food and Drug Administration. 1994. 21 CFR Part 101, Food labeling: Nutrient content claims, general principles; health claims, general requirements and other specific requirements for individual health claims. Docket 94P-0390, p. 66208.

U.S. Food and Drug Administration. 1999. May. The food label. Retrieved March 1, 2001. http://www.fda.gov/opacom/backgrounders/foodlabel/newlabel.html

Villas, James. 1982. *American taste*. New York: Arbor House.

Vinson, Joe A., and Barbara A. Hontz. 1995. Phenol antioxidant index: Comparative antioxidant effectiveness of red and white wines. *Journal of Agricultural and Food Chemistry*, 43, pp. 401–403.

Visser, Margaret. 1995. *The rituals of dinner*. Toronto, Canada: HarperCollins Publishers.

War Food Administration. 1942. *Proceedings of the National Nutrition Conference for Defense, May 26–28, 1941*. Washington: Government Printing Office.

Warde, Alan. 1997. *Consumption, food and taste*. Thousand Oaks, CA: Sage Publications.

Waterhouse, Andrew L. 1994, July. It could be the phenolic antioxidants, stupid. *Wines and Vines*, 75, pp. 38–42.

Watson, James. 1997. *Golden arches east: McDonald's in East Asia*. Stanford, CA: Stanford University Press.

Watson, James, and Melissa Caldwell, eds. 2005. *The cultural politics of food and eating: A reader*. Malden, MA: Blackwell Publishing.

Weaver, Richard. 1995. *The ethics of rhetoric*. Washington, DC: LEA.

Weismantel, M. J. 1988. *Food, gender and poverty in the Ecuadorian Andes*. Philadelphia: University of Pennsylvania Press.

Welsh, Susan O., et al. 1993. *USDA's food guide: Background and development*. USDA misc. publication no. 1514.

Welsh, Susan, C. Davis, and A. Shaw. 1992, November/December. Development of the Food Guide Pyramid. *Nutrition Today*, p. 7.

Welsh, Susan. 1994. Atwater to present: Evolution of nutrition information. *Journal of Nutrition*, 124, pp. 1800–1801S.

Wiebe, Robert. 1967. *The search for order: 1877–1920*. New York: Hill and Wang.

Wiggen, Jeanne. 1993. The room calorimeter: Atwater's "copper box" revisited. *Agricultural Research*, 41, pp. 12–14.

Wilder, Russell M. 1941. *Nutrition, the armor of robust health*. Washington, DC: Government Printing Office.

Willett, Walter C. 2001. *Eat, drink, and be healthy: The Harvard Medical School guide to healthy eating*. New York: Simon and Schuster.

Wise, Norton, ed. 1995. *The values of precision*. Princeton: Princeton University Press.

Witt, Doris. 1999. *Black hunger: Food and the politics of U.S. identity*. New York: Oxford University Press.

Wolf, I. D., and B. B. Peterkin. 1984, July. Dietary guidelines: The USDA perspective. *Food Technology*, 38, pp. 80–86.

Woolf, Harry Ed. 1961. *Quantification: A history of measurement in the natural and social sciences*. Indianapolis: Bobbs-Merrill Company.

Ziman, John. 1978. *Reliable knowledge: An exploration of the grounds for belief in science*. Cambridge: Cambridge University Press.

Websites and Authorless Publications

1991–2001 prevalence of obesity among U.S. adults by state. 2003, November 17. U.S. Department of Health and Human Services. Retrieved from http://www.cdc.gov/nccdphp/dnpa/obesity/trend/prev_reg.htm.

Ark of taste and presidia, www.slowfood.com/eng/sf_arca_presidi/sf_arca.lasso. Retrieved February 18, 2003, ed. John Irving.

Chez Panisse. www.chezpanisse.com. Retrieved March 2003.

Chowhound. www.chowhound.com. Retrieved multiple times, December 2003.

The French Paradox. 1991, November 17. Narr. Mike Wallace. *60 Minutes*. CBS.

"French paradox" revisits America as CardioFlav 500. 2000, June. *Health Products Business*, 46, p. 52.

Le *Beaujolais* eternal est arrive. 1997, March 10. *Forbes*. p. 90.

A little "lite" reading, ed. USFDA. Retrieved March 10, 2001 from www.fda.gov/fdac/special/foodlabel/lite.html

Lot to be said for local produce. 2002. August. *Dairy Farmer*, p. 6

Master of food, http://www.slowfood.com/eng/sf_master/sf_master_corsi.lasso. Retrieved March 2, 2003, ed. John Irving.

Tasting notes. 2003 April. *Slow*, p. 101.

U.S. puts wine health label on hold. 2000, January. *Beverage Industry*, 91, p. 9.

Università di Scienze Gastronomiche. 2003. Bra: Commission of the University of Gastronomic Sciences.

University of Gastronomic sciences. http://www.slowfood.com/eng/sf_universita/sf_universita.lasso. Retrieved March 15, 2003, ed. John Irving.

Index

DATE DUE

DEMCO, INC. 38-2931